INDIAN MEDICAL SCIENCE SERIES—No. 3

# Clinical Application of Ayurvedic Remedies

## AND

## A List of Ayurvedic Preparations

*By*

**A PANEL OF VAIDYAS**

**SRI SATGURU PUBLICATIONS**

**DELHI—INDIA**

*Published by :*
Sri Satguru Publications
*A Division of :*
Indian Books Centre
Indological and Oriental Publishers
40/5, Shakti Nagar,
Delhi-110007
(INDIA)

Second Edition; Delhi 1986
Third Edition; Delhi 1994
Fourth Edition - Delhi - 1998

ISBN - 81 - 7030 - 101 - 7

Published by Sunil Gupta for Sri Satguru Publications a division of Indian Books Centre, 40/5, Shakti Nagar, Delhi-110 007, India and printed at Mudran Bharti, Delhi-110007

# CONTENTS.

# PREFACE.

In preparing this brochure we are actuated by two motives. We intend in the first place, to supply to our native physicians a sort of guide in their profession. The original works of Ayurvedic medicine are in Sanscrit ; there are very few reliable translations of these works. Again the order of arrangement in these works is such that one could not get a complete treatment of any one particular subject in any one work. Owing to this and many other reasons, our native physicians are in great want of such a guide book.

In the second place, many doctors have latterly taken to the use of our native drugs, either out of respect to our old Ayurved or because their patients demand them. These doctors have no time to study the Sanscrit texts of Ayurvedic medicine and their scientific training does not allow them to make experiments on human lives, of drugs about which they know nothing definite. Our aim is to supply this information of the Shastric method of using native drugs to our respected clientele of this class.

In order to fulfil both these aims at the same time, we have made the use of the comparative method. At first sight, it may appear impossible to institute a comparison between the old Ayurveda developed by the ancient Rishis more than two thousand years ago, and the system of European medicine that is being developed at such rapid strides in this age of scientific progress. But a slight reflection will help to dispell such pessimistic ideas. It has to be remembered that the basis of both the systems is 'experience.' Western medicine has certainly taken very rapid strides in Anatomy, Physiology, &c., because we possess to-day instruments for very minute and accurate observations, such as were not even dreamt of in those days. Hence the physiology of Ayurveda based on mere outward observation, has no lessons to teach to the new physiology studied with the help of the most elaborate instruments. But treatment is chiefly a subject of experience, and it is probable that in this broad expanses of India, the Rishis may have derived an extended experience of many diseases. So that in this sphere, it is possible to use the method of comparison. We may make this a little more clear by an example or two. Doctors recommend in high fever some kind of cold treatment. Ayurveda also recommends the same. "*Dividing fevers into cold and hot*, such treatment as cold bath, application of some cooling substance, or dripping some cold liquid continuously for a long time should be used, as may be necessary." *Charaka.* Again, "physicians treat diseases due to heat by cold producing agents." (*Ibid.*) Thus Ayurvedic and European medicines are at one in recommending cold treatment in the heat of fevers. It is natural that the particular substance recommended for inducing cold will be different in the different cases. The old Rishis used Chandan-sandal, lotus, cold water, &c.; to-day we can get ice in plenty and so use it; but the basic principle of both is the same, *viz*:—induce cold and lower temperature in the heat of fever.

Sushruta recommends surgery in dropsy, stone, cancer, intestinal obstruction, &c. European medicine also recommends surgery in these cases. The treatment of snake bite in both systems is the same, *viz*: to open the wound and cauterise it. To stop vomiting, doctors recommend sucking ice: Charaka recommends very 'cold' water. The ancient Aryans used bael fruit in cases of dysentery two thousand years ago, and to-day the doctor recommends the same. Such instances may be extended to an enormous length. Discriminating readers will thus be able to see that in the treatment of diseases, it is not difficult to compare the East with the West. How far the comparison given in this pamphlet has been justified can only be determined by learned physicians and eminent doctors after somewhat extended experience. This is a first attempt in this direction, and as such, is bound to have many defects. We shall be highly obliged if doctors and Vaidyas will help us to weed out its defects by suggestions and improvements.

In preparing this brochure, we have freely drawn upon the inexhaustible store given to us by the ancient Rishis. We have taken prescriptions from Charaka, Sushruta, Vriddha,

Vag Bhatta, Ashtang hridaya, Rasa hridaya, Sharangdhar, Bhavprakash, Rasa Ratna Samuchchaya, Yoga Ratnakar, Bhaishajya Ratnavali, Nighant Ratnaker, &c., and for symptoms of diseases, we have also consulted Madhav Nidan. For comparison with Western medicine, we have used Moore's Family Medicine, Du la Foy's Practice of Medicine, Robert's Practice of Medicine, Vhitla's Dictionary of Treatment, Sharir by Dr. T. M. Shah, &c. For the English equivalents of the Sanskrit names of diseases, we have taken the help of Dr. Garde's Marathi rendering of Madhav Nidan, and the Madhav Nidan with commentary, 4th Edn., published by the Nirnaya Sagar Press, Bombay. We have also made some use of the list of Wellcome, Abbot, Park Davis, &c. Over and above these, we have also drawn upon the practical experience of a very high order. The proprietor of this concern has inherited a very widely extended medical practice, and he has a wide experience of Western and Eastern methods of treatment, which has been used in the preparation of this work. Several kind friends have also given us the benefit of their experience and learning, among whom we must mention Vaidraj Vishvanath Vithalji, State Physician to H. H. the Thakore Saheb of Morvi, Vaid Jadavji Tricumji Acharya, editor of Ayurvedic Granthmala, Vaidraj Prabhulal Prabhashanker, Vaidraj Amritlal Pranshanker. Another kind friend Dr. S. K. Vaidya, L.M. & S., has gone through the conspectus of diseases from beginning to end. Our best thanks are due to these gentlemen for their suggestions. In Bombay, this city of multi-sided activities and interests, consultations between doctors and Vaidyas are of ordinary occurrence, and if at such times, this small brochure helps both of them to understand each other better than before, we shall consider our pains to have been well taken.

This digest is made up of three divisions. (1) An index of diseases, (2) an index of medicines, and (3) miscellaneous information for Vaidyas. The index of diseases is alphabetically arranged, and an index of their Sanskrit names is given at the end. So that one can easily find the treatment of any disease, if one knows either its English or Sanskrit name. In the second division, decoctions, powders, pills, tablets, confections, &c., are shown separately, and then under each heading, the medicines are arranged alphabetically; so that if any one knows whether a particular drug is a pill or decoction or powder, he can find it out at once under its proper heading. For others, there is also a general index of all the drugs at the end. In the third division, we have given hints as to the general regimen in different cases, urine examination, tables of weights and measures, &c.

In the medical guides nowadays it has become customary to give general hints as to temperance in the satisfaction of the appetites when prescribing various medicines for diseases. But diet has relation with disease and not with medicine. It is true that in some very hot medicines like marking nuts, some particular things are especially prohibited, *e.g.*, when marking nuts are being taken, capsicum and even exposure to the sun leads to eruptions. But such drugs are few and far between, and even in their case, if taken in proper dose, there is not much danger. But in some diseases, diet has a special significance, *e.g.*, diabetics pass sugar in their urine, hence they should avoid in their food, sugar or any other substances which generally are transformed into sugar. Thus diet has a special relation with diseases and in some cases is a very important element in the treatment of diseases, but ordinary general hints are a useless burden on the patient. In this brochure, we have given in a separate chapter only those hints as to diet, which according to the above rule, are necessary in the various diseases, and some special hints in the use of particular medicines like marking nuts, have been given in short, in the section dealing with these drugs. Such general remarks that "temperance in the satisfaction of bodily appetites preserves health, and want of it brings on disease," are principles of ordinary health and should not be confounded with dietetics. It is needless for example, when prescribing a particular drug, to advise avoidance of over-eating; over-eating is bad in all cases, and does not need a special precaution in any particular disease.

## Dose.

The doses prescribed herein are only general and will require modification, in particulaı cases. The dose depends upoıı the condition of the patient, the stage of the disease, the age of the patient, his habits, &c. Vagbhatta says in Ashtang Kalpa Ch. VI. "There is no general rule as to the dose; the dose must be determined by a consideration of the disease, the constitution of the patient, his strength, his age, the character of the country and time." Modern Vaidyas do not stick to the old regulation of the Shastras—of prescribing 4 tolas; buy they have modified it to suit modern times. We also have given the usual doses to be 5 to 20 grains, 1 to 4 pills, 1 to 4 tolas, &c.—in the ratıo of 1 to 4. So that 1 represents the minimum and 4 the maximum dose for an average adult. We have not indicated separate doses for children, but in a general table, indicated the usual modifications for ages 1 month to 21 years; so that from the dose for adults, a man may determine the dose suitable to his age. Some useful hints as to the dose and the effects of particular drugs are also given in the third part.

Drugs have to be taken in different media. In some lists are found half a dozen drugs prescribed as media for taking a particular drug. It is true that one sometimes has to prescribe a mixture for a particular disease, but that is because each ingredient has a certain relation to the disease, and not because it has any relation with the other drugs prescribed. In the index of diseases, we have already stated what mixtures are to be prescribed in different diseases; we have also stated in the proper places whether a drug should be taken in a decoction, honey, Ghrita, milk, sugar or water; when nothing is stated, simple water is the medium.

## Urine Examination.

The diagnosis of certain diseases is confirmed by urine examination. Hence we have also devoted a short chapter to that subject. The importance of this subject has been established definitely in European medicine. Hence we have taken from that science that much amount of information about the subject as may enable our ordinary Vaidyas to make urine examination with the help of ordinary materials.

## References.

In the index of diseases, under the Sanskrit names of diseases, we have given the reference to the original work in which a full treatment of the particular disease is given. For those diseases, which are rather difficult to diagnose at first sight, we have given their symptoms also. These symptoms we have adopted from Moore's Family Medicine, Du la Foy's Practice of Medicine, and Dr. T. M. Shah's Sharir; but we have not been able to make special references in each case, and so make this general statement here. The symptoms, &c., have been taken from English works of medicine in preference to the old Sanskrit works, simply because in the Sanskrit works, the symptoms are so few, that it requires a competent Vaidya of wide experience to apply the diagnosis; while in European medicine, the symptoms given are very extended, so that the difficulty of diagnosis is very much lightened. We have compared the two systems and satisfied ourselves that the difference between the two systems is only one of conciseness and diffusion; though to attempt to prove that point here, would take us far beyond the limits of this small brochure.

The treatment prescribed by us is also based on the Ayurveda; here and there, we have stuck to the letter or merely adapted the substance; hence, we have not been able to indicate every source for the treatment prescribed.

In the index of medicines, a very few are special preparations invented by us. The rest are all derived from Shastras, and in their case we have indicated the source from which we have taken the prescription. So that drugs for which no reference is given is to be understood as our special preparation. For preparations of Ayurvedic medicines, we have literally followed the authorities which have been indicated..

Several Bhasmas and Rasayanas prepared in the Rasa Shala at Jamnagar have been indicated by a distinct reference to that effect.

The question of dietetics is treated according to the principles of Western medicine, but it does not contravene our Ayurvedic principles.

# PART I.

## Clinical Application of Ayurvedic Remedies.

### ABORTION. *GARBHAPAT.* S. Sha. Ch. 10. Ch. Sha. Ch. 8.

*THREATENED*—Perfect quiet and rest in a cool room. Dadimivati and Vasavaleha followed by Saurashtraja solution (1 tablet in 1 oz. of water) after an interval of 4 hours.

*INEVITABLE*—To prevent profuse loss of blood, Saurashtraja Solution (1 tablet in 1 oz. of water) with Vasavaleha, should be given.

*LOCALLY*—Clothes saturated with cold water should be applied to the external outlet in threatened abortion.

*AFTER TREATMENT*—Rest in bed. Bowels should be maintained moderately open by castor oil or Swadishta virechana. Tonic pills or Agnitundi pills after meals.

*DIET*—Simple.

---

### ABSCESS. *VIDRADHI.* S. Ni. Ch. 9. Ch. Su. Ch. 19.

To prevent formation of matter, Dashang lepa or lotion of Shital tikdi should be applied on the part affected. The part should be kept in perfect rest and in an elevated position as much as possible. But if matter has formed already, to further the ripening and pointing of the abscess hot fomentations, poultices and Doshaghna lepa should be applied on the part. If the pain is severe, hot fomentations with poppy head water or Datura leaves will give relief.

*INTERNALLY*—Samudraka virechana once in the beginning and Samshamani pills three times a day to be continued for some time. Even after incision or bursting, poultices should be continued for a short time. (See Ulcer).

*CHRONIC*—General debility, anæmia, scrofula, etc., should be corrected as indicated under those headings.

## ACNE. *YOUVANPITKA.* S. Ni. Ch. 8.

Treat indigestion and insist on regular exercise; free bowel action and simple diet, with no fatty foods nor excessive quantities of tea. Cold bath, rubbing with a rough towel and strict cleanliness will prevent acne as a rule.

*INTERNALLY*—Samudraka virechana in the beginning and then Saptamrit with Manjishthadi quath.

*LOCALLY*—Wash with hot water and rub with a rough towel. If the part is inflamed, foment only. Express comedones. Apply Vachadi lepa or Kustumbarvadi lepa and Manjishthadi oil, Haridradi oil or Kanaka oil, which are useful applications after the part has been thoroughly washed.

---

## ACIDITY. *AMLAPITTA.* Ch. Su. Ch. 2. Ma. Ni.

Is a frequent symptom of indigestion and often accompanies chronic rheumatism and gout. When acidity is slight, the symptoms are limited to heart-burn, flatulence or to a little acid rising and sour eructations. There may be also fulness, oppression, uneasiness, or even aching pain felt in the chest. In larger quantity, acidity causes irregularity or capriciousness of appetite, head-ache, aching of the limbs, sleeplessness, depression of spirits, nausea, pain at the pit of the stomach, and skin affections.

*TREATMENT*—Consists in avoiding those articles of diet which produce acidity, *e.g.* unripe fruit, cabbage, sugar and food containing much starch, as rice, potatoes, arrowroot, etc.

*INTERNALLY*—Avipatyakara with Swarjika or Shiva-kshar-pachan in the morning; Agnitundi vati after meals. If dyspeptic, give Sudarshana churna or Amritadi quath in the morning with Swarjika kshara (see Heart-burn). Cocoanut water should be given to drink.

---

## AFTER-PAINS. *MAKKAL.* S. Sha. Ch. 10.

Naturally after-pains are beneficial and therefore need no treatment; but if found troublesome, give Akarkarbhadi with Karpasmul quath and Devdarvadi quath with Pippalyadi churna.

**ALBUMINURIA.** *LALAMEHA.* Ch. Chi. Ch. 6.

(See Examination of urine) also see (Diet tables and general directions).

Treat the primary cause, *e. g.* Heart disease, Nephritis, etc. In the beginning give Eliyakadi pills at night and Samudraka virechana in the morning; then Chandraprabha pills or Mehamudgar rasa every morning and evening, and Trikatuadi pills with Agnitundi after meals.

---

**ALCOHOLISM.** *MADATYAYA.* S. U. Ch. 47. Ch. Chi. Ch. 12.

Prohibit alcohol absolutely and order abundant food. Hot air baths or hot water baths with massage are beneficial.

For gastro-intestinal catarrh Akarkarbhadi or Jatiphaladi churna with Guduchyadi quath morning and evening; Ashtang lavana with meals and Narsinha churna after meals.

---

**AMENORRHŒA.** *ARTAV-DOSH* Ch.Chi. Ch. 30. *KSHINARTAV* S. Sha. Ch. 2.

Treat the cause—(*e.g.* often dependent on anæmia). If it be mechanical, consult some expert of women diseases.

*INTERNALLY*—Kashisadi pills are the best. If constipative, give Hingu-eliyadi or Eliyadi pills.

Mustard hip bath.

---

**ANÆMIA.** *PANDU-ROGA.* S. U. Ch. 44. Ch. Chi. Ch. 20.

(See Diet tables and general directions).

In the beginning and afterwards also, when bowels appear costive, give Trivritadi churna or Swadishta virechana daily, Arogyavardhani pills with Sudarshana morning and evening, and Mandurvatak, Punarnava mandura or Narayan jwarankusha after meals. For children who eat earth, prescribe Mandura-vatak with Samshamani and Harde water.

*SECONDARY*—Treat the cause: *e.g.* hæmorrhage, leucorrhœa, syphilis, malaria, tubercle, lead, mercury or arsenic poisoning, chronic constipation, etc.

**ANGINA PECTORIS.** ***HRADGRAHA HRAD-ROGA.*** S. Ni. Ch 1. Ch. Chi. Ch. 26.

*SYMPTOMS*—The disease is characterised by paroxysms of pain, faintness, difficulty of breathing, and anxiety amounting to terror at times. It is most common among men and rarely attacks persons under 40 years of age.

The first paroxysm may occur after some violent exertion or when the patient is walking uphill, or after a heavy meal. The attack is very likely to recur, but at no fixed interval—months or years sometimes elapsing.

Improve general health ; treat gout if present.

To prevent future attacks. Greatest care should be taken in diet and all exertion which accelerates breathing should be avoided. Anand Bhairav with Kakubhadi Churna may be given twice a day.

*DURING ATTACK*—Jatiphaladi or Krimi Kuthara Rasa should be given in small doses frequently.

If the attack comes after a hearty meal, Madanadi Vaman as an emetic will probably give relief. Samudraka Virechana may be given as a purgative if the bowels are confined.

*LOCALLY*—Fomentations of hot water or mustard poultice on the chest.

(*The best remedy in alopathy is Amyl Nitrite which should be inhaled during attack*).

---

**ANOREXIA.** ***AROCHAK.*** S. U. Ch. 57. Ch. Chi. Ch. 26.

If due to constipation give Shiva-kshar-pachan ; if dyspeptic, give Agnitundi vati after meals, and Guduchyadi quath or Sudarshana with Swarjikakshara morning and evening.

To make food agreeable, Hingu-ashtak churna, Saindhavadi, Dadimashtak or Yawani khandav churna with or before meals.

Agreeable food, sea-bath, and other exercises are beneficial.

---

**APHONIA.** ***MOOKATVA.*** S. Ni. Ch. 1. Ch. Su. Ch. 20.

Locate and treat the cause.

Praval bhasma with Yavakshara and Saraswat ghrita or Brahmi ghrita in the morning, and Saptamrit with Agnitundi vati after meals.

*DIET*—Nutritious, Chyavanprasha avaleh with milk.

---

## APHTHÆ. *SARVASARMUKH-ROGA*. S. Ni. Ch. 16.

*SYMPTOMS*—This disease consists of an eruption on the tongue, lips, cheek and gums, of small white vesicles, which discharge whitish mucus. This mucus adheres for some days ; and then falling off, discloses small ulcers.

If the child is teething and the gums are swollen, they should be lanced.

If the bowels are costive, castor oil or Samudraka virechana should be given. But in case of diarrhœa, Arkadi churna and Samshamani pills are effective. If there is debility, Mandura vatak and Samshamani pills are effective.

*LOCALLY*—Jantughna and Grahi tikdi one in 1 oz. of honey should be applied in the mouth twice or thrice daily.

It is better to feed a child with mother's breast ; but if the child is fed by hand, milk should be diluted with lime water.

*FOR ADULTS*—Only milk diet is the best treatment.

---

## APOPLEXY. *SANYAS*. S, U. Ch. 46.

Is usually ultimately characterised by insensibility, accompanied by slow, noisy, puffing breathing and frothy saliva about the mouth. The teeth are clenched and the person is unable to swallow. The countenance becomes flushed or livid ; the eyes are dull and glassy, the mouth is drawn to one side, the limbs are motionless and rigid, but sometimes convulsed often only on one side of the body. The bowels are either obstinately confined or motions are passed involuntarily ; the same may be said of urine. The duration of an apopletic fit varies from 2 to 3 hours or as many days.

Apoplexy requires to be distinguished from fainting from the effects of alcohol, from the results of narcotic poisons such as opium, and from epilepsy.

*FAINTING*—Occurs principally to young, nervous or hysterical women; apoplexy to elderly people. As a rule, persons fainting recover in a few minutes. The apopletic attack continues for many hours.

Apoplexy is best distinguished from effects of alcohol by the history of the case; by the smell of liquor in the person's breath.

In the drunken fit, the pupils are equal; while in apoplexy, one is often contracted and the other dilated.

Apoplexy is best distinguished from poisoning by opium, by history of the case, by the absence or presence of the smell of opium in the breath or vomit. In apoplexy the patient cannot be roused; while in opium poisoning, he may generally be roused easily.

Apoplexy is known from epilepsy by the presence of puffing breathing, which is absent in the latter malady. In epilepsy, the eyes are turned up under the lids, so that the whites are only visible, and the person generally falls down with a loud cry, none of which is present in epilepsy.

*TREATMENT*—Perfect rest and quiet. The head and shoulders should be propped towards the right side; the patient should not be troubled with medicines or anything else. Cold water (ice) or lotion of Shitala Tikdi should be applied to the forehead. The patient may be drawn down gently towards the foot of the bed until the knees being bent, the legs hang over. The feet should be kept in hot water for about ten minutes, after which bottles filled with hot water should be applied to them. The mustard poultices should be allowed to remain on the calves for an hour. Leeches or venesection is sometimes necessary. If the bladder is full, urine should be drawn off with catheter, and fomentations applied over loins. As soon as the patient can swallow, one drop of croton oil may be given: if oil is not at hand, one or two croton seeds, or Naracha rasa. Cold water draughts to drink. An Asafœtida enema should be given as soon as possible.

*DURING CONVALESCENCE*—Ashva Kanchuki or Samudraka Virechan in the morning and Agnitundi after meals. For habitual patients, simple habits, low diet, and Samudraka Virechana with Chandraprabha, when necessary.

---

## ASCITES. *JALODAR.* S. Ni. Ch. 7. Ch. Chi. Ch. 18.

(See Dropsy).

Dropsy of the Peritoneum is called Jalodar. Operation of tapping done in the early stage may prolong life.

---

## ASTHMA. *SHWAS (TAMAKA.)* S. U. Ch. 51. Ch. Chi. Ch. 21.

*AVOID*—Exciting causes, places, foods or occupations likely to induce attack.

*TREAT*—Pulmonary, cardiac, gastro-intestinal, renal and other disorders, including any abnormal conditions of the nose or throat. Never exceed in diet, avoid late dinners, do not allow constipation or indigestion to occur.

Medicines preventive of an attack are:—Eliyakadi at night and Samudraka virechana next morning twice a week. Samshamani pills morning and evening with Sudarshana and Swarjika kshar, and Agnitundi Vati with Mandur-loha after meals for debility.

*DIET*—Milk with Chyavanprash Avaleha.

*DURING ATTACK*—In the beginning, hot coffee with little or no sugar, or Swarjika kshara in a large dose. Madanadi Vaman if the attack has followed an injudicious meal. Then if the fit is not very severe, Shwaskuthara with Harade avaleha or Vasavaleha. When it is too severe, Jatiphaladi should be given every hour in small doses. If relief is not obtained after two doses of

Jatiphaladi, Dadimi vati should be tried in small doses. If there is much coughing, Agnirasa should be given with Vasaraga.

Inhalation of steam or of Shwasghna churna, or smoking of Shwasghna dhumravarti.

*LOCALLY.*—Poultice on the chest and fomentation on the back.

*DIET.*—Hot milk.

---

## BITES & STINGS. *DANSHA.* S. Ka. Ch. 3-5-6. Ch. Chi. Ch. 25.

### Mouse-bite—

*LOCALLY*—Remove the sting. Rub it with Tutha tikdi. Apply Shirishadi lepa over the part.

*INTERNALLY*—Madanadi-vamana as an emetic and Ichhabhedi as a purgative.

### Snake-bite—

*LOCALLY*—Ligature the part above the bite; incise margins of the wound, suck the wound, and rub in ¼ gr. Rasakarpura or Dalchikna. Pour water on the head.

### Scorpion-bite—

*LOCALLY*—Surashtraja lotion should be applied on the part affected.

---

## BLEPHARITIS. *PAKSHMASHAT.* V. U. Ch. 8.

A number of little styes or pustules form at the roots of eyelashes. They discharge a yellowish fluid, which mats the eyelashes together. There is considerable smarting and itching, and often overflow of tears. The eyelashes may be lost. The malady is most common in children affected by a scrofulous taint.

The eyelashes should be frequently washed with Surashtraja Solution (1 tablet of 5 grs. in 2 ozs. of water) or Kasis tikdi Solution (1 in 1 oz. water). Jasata ointment may be applied to the eyelids with a feather at night.

*INTERNALLY*—Saptamrit Churna with milk.

---

**BOILS.** *PITIKA.* S. Ni. Ch. 6. Ch. Su. Ch. 18.

Examine urine for sugar. If found, treat as Diabetes.

*INTERNALLY*—Trivritadi Churna or Samudraka Virechana, as a purgative. If drastic purgative is required, Ichhabhedi may be given. After that any one or more of the following may be given with good effect: Kishora Guggula, Amritadi Guggula, or Devkusumadi with Amritadi quath or Manjisthadi quath and Swarjika-kshar.

*LOCALLY*—Fomentations with hot water or poultice, or Doshaghna lepa should be applied to the part affected. Parvativilasa Taila or Datura leaves to be applied to lessen pain.

*DIET*—Vegetables may be taken with advantage. (See Ulcer).

---

**BRONCHITIS.** *KASBHEDA (COUGH-JANYA.)* S. U. Ch. 52. Ch. Chi. Ch. 22

Bronchitis is generally caused by chill, and commences with symptoms of a common cold.

There is first running at the nose and a feeling of chilliness and aching pains in the limbs; slight rise of temperature; the patient is feverish and thirsty, and there is languor, headache, furred tongue, loss of appetite and restlessness. There is also a feeling of soreness behind the breast bone and of constriction or tightness of the chest. At first there is a dry, hacking cough, the breathing is oppressed and difficult, and very little phlegm is brought up. The fever often becomes considerable, and the pulse may rise to 120 or higher. In three or four days the cough becomes looser and the expectoration more abundant.

Throughout the attack, wheezing sounds may be heard with the breathing and a thrill may be felt when the hand is placed on the chest or back.

*TREATMENT*—Hot bath, hot foot bath, light food, hot Shunthi quath, milk, tea or coffee to drink. Protection from draughts and cold. Rest in bed. Linseed poultices on the chest.

In the beginning Samudraka virechana to open the bowels. During the whole illness, Vasavaleha, Agni rasa with Kantakari avaleha or Vasaraga, and Harade avaleha should be given for free expectoration everyday whenever necessary. For troublesome cough and restlessness, Jatifaladi, Kanaka sunder or arkadi may be given.

In chronic cases, Krimikuthara with Arkadi quath is beneficial. Yashtiadi pills to be kept in the mouth and allowed to be dissolved slowly. For severe cough, Agni rasa or Vasaraga with Swarjika kshara, twice daily; and Sitopaladi or Talisadi may be given after meals. Treat dyspepsia: teach deep respiration.

## BRONCHITIS OF CHILDREN.

The acute bronchitis of children is generally of graver importance than when the disease attacks the adult. The attack is generally due to cold.

*TREATMENT*—Keep the child indoors, maintain the temperature of the room equable. Great relief will be found by moistening the atmosphere by allowing steam to pass into the room through a boiling kettle or even an ordinary cooking vessel. Great care must be taken to prevent cold draughts. Further measures, if necessary, are in applying to the chest a large piece of thick flannel soaked in hot water. This may be continued 24 to 36 hours till relief is found. The bowels, if confined, should be acted upon by castor oil. If there is much wheezing or stuffing of the chest, Arka churna or Madanadivaman churna once daily as an emetic. During the whole illness, Agnirasa, Shringyadi Churna or Vishadi churna twice a day should be administered. Even after cure, the child should be protected from cold.

## BUBO. *BRAGHNA.* Ch. Su. Ch. 18. Ma. Ni.

Rest in the horizontal position. If due to syphilis, treat syphilis.

*INTERNALLY*—Samudraka virechana in the beginning: if drastic purgative is required use Ichhabhedi: then Amrita guggula and Punarnavadi quath daily.

*LOCALLY*—Cold lotion of Shitlal tikadi or Dashang lepa should be applied to prevent formation of matter, and Vishagarbha taila as an anodyne. But if formation becomes unavoidable, apply fomentations of hot water or poultices and Doshaghna lepa, and treat as an abscess.

---

## BURNING OF THE FEET. *PADA-DAHA* S. Ni. Ch. 1.

*LOCALLY*—Apply oil of Sesamum or Chandanadi taila; bathing the feet in strong saline solution should be tried. Sea-bath is also beneficial.

*INTERNALLY*—Samudraka virechana in the beginning, Samshamani pills morning and evening. and Saptamrit with Agnitundi or tonic pills after meals. If there is sleeplessness, give Jatiphaladi at night.

---

## CALCULI BILIARY, Or Gall Stones, *ASHMARI (Pittatmak)*

Gall stones are small substances which form by the deposit in the gall-bladder of certain elements of the bile. So long as the stone remains in the gall-bladder, it does not produce any inconvenience. The flow of bile sometimes carries a small stone into the short duct of tube leading from the gall bladder into the intestines without causing any pain. But a large stone causes sudden attacks of shivering and excruciating pain, immediately to the right of the pit of the stomach shooting to the back with vomiting first of the contents of the stomach and then of sour bile. There is occasionally sudden jaundice. In the absence of bile, the stools will be clay coloured.

During attack, gall stone can be distinguished from Gravel by the following symptoms:—

| *Gravel (Stone in the Kidney).* | *Gall Stone.* |
|---|---|
| Pain in loins : usually on one side. | Not. |
| Pain shooting from loins down the groin and thighs. | Pain to right of pit of stomach shooting to the back. |
| On either side, rarely both. | Pain most on right side. |
| Numbness of thigh or leg. | Not. |
| Testicles drawn up. | Not. |
| Frequent desire to make water. | Not. |
| Making water may be painful. | Not. |
| Water scanty, high coloured or bloody. | Not altered. |
| Previous history of gravel, gout, or rheumatism. | Previous history of gall stone jaundice and pale 'stool.' |
| Most common in men. | Most common in women. |
| Begins in middle age. | Rare under 50 years of age. |

*PREVENTION*—Of recurrence of the stone: Regular diet and exercise : give abundant fluid such as tea, etc. Samudraka virechana as purgative when necessary. Swarjika, Yavakshar or Chandraprabha three times daily and Sesamum oil 4 to 8 ozs. every day.

*DURING ATTACK*—Hot bath. Hot fomentations over the paining part.

*INTERNALLY*—If the attack comes on after a full meal, Madanadi Vaman as an emetic ; otherwise a tumbler of hot water with Sarjika-kshara. If the bowels are costive, Samudraka virechana in a large dose and head-ache cure as an anodyne.

---

## GRAVEL, *SHARKARA.* S. U. Ch. 59. Ch. Chi. Ch. 26.
## Calculi Renal.

No stimulants. Between attacks, give internally Chandraprabha and Gokshur guggula or Gokshuradyavaleha with Virtarvadi quath, or Gokshuradi Churna with milk morning and evening. When the urine is acid and bowels costive, Sudarshana

Churna with Swarjika Kshara and Samudraka Virechana combined, three hours after the principal meals; or Yavakshara alone, as long as urine remains acid.

During fit of Gravel: The patient should be placed in a hot bath and fomentations applied over the loins. Internally Dadimivati.

*DIET*—Sugar, coffee, butter, cream, &c., should be avoided. A tumbler of hot water three times a day. Barley or Linseed water should be taken plentifully.

---

## CALCULI (Urinary) *ASHMARI.* S. Chi. Ch. 7. Ch. Chi. Ch 26.

No stimulants. Between attacks, give—

*INTERNALLY*:—Chandraprabha, Gokshura Guggula or Gokshuradi—Avaleha with Virtarvadi Quath morning and evening and Yavakshara three hours after the principal meal.

For diet and local treatment during attack see Calculi Renal.

Operation is sometimes necessary.

---

## CANCER. *MANSARBUD.* S. Ni. Ch. 14.

Cancer may occur in any part of the body, but it is most common in the breasts of women, the lips, the skin, the stomach, the testicle, the tongue and the womb. It is often a hereditary disease.

Cancerous growths are very liable to fatty degeneration. All cancerous growths tend to ulcerate; the ulcers having no disposition to heal, but being inclined to spread. Pain and tenderness are very severe, the pain being frequently of lancinating or burning character. General symptoms are: a peculiar sallow cachetic look, with a yellowish earthy tint of countenance; a careworn, gloomy expression, debility and languor which may culminate in a feeling of extreme depression and exhaustion; anæmia and its accompaniments and irregular fever.

This disease is curable by knife only. (*Sushruta ch* 25.) Akarkarbhadi; Jatiphaladi and Kanaka Sundar are useful as anodyne. Warm enema of Tankan-Amla (boric acid) in cancer of rectum does much relief.

## CARBUNCLE. *VINATA PRAMEHA PITAKA.*

S. Ni. Ch. 6.
Ch. Su. Ch. 19.

Examine carefully for cause.

Examine urine for sugar.

*INTERNALLY.*—Samudraka Virechana as an aperient in the beginning. Then for fever and debility, Samshamani with Kiratadi Quath morning and evening and Lohe Bhasma with Pravai Bhasma and Sitopaladi after meals. If the patient is diabetic, add Dadimivati after meals and Swarjikakshar morning and evening.

*LOCALLY.*—Doshaghna Lepa or hot poultice to be applied. As soon as carbuncle forms matter, free crucial incision should be made; and all the decayed matter should be removed; and the part should be dressed with Jatyadi malam when the discharge ceases. By Alopathic doctors at first the cavity is usually swabbed with carbolic acid one part and glycerine 5 parts.

## CHICKEN-POX.

Insist on simple and milk diet and confinement to one room with proper hygiene. Stop itching.

*INTERNALLY.*—As a mild purgative Samudraka Virechana or Ashwa Kanchuki: To control fever give Tribhuvankirti with Parpat decoction; if diuretic is required give Chandraprabha. Prescribe Samshamani daily.

*LOCALLY.*—Snigdha Malama to be applied to allay itching. The same ointment should be applied after the scabs have fallen off.

## CHLOROSIS. *PANDU-ROGA* S. U. Ch. 44. Ch. Chi. Ch. 20.

When Anæmia is connected with the first appearance or irregularities of the monthly courses of women, it is often called *Chlorosis.*

Give Dhatri-Avaleha morning and evening and Narayan Jwarankush after meals.

For further treatment, see Anæmia.

If disorders of monthly flow exist, the treatment of ammenorrhœa or dysmennorhœa should be pursued. Moderate exercise, free ventilation, and nourishing diet are beneficial.

## CHOLERA. *VISHOOCHIKA.* S. U. Ch. 56. Ch. Vi. Ch. 2.

Rest in bed.

First evacuate the stomach with 2 or 3 doses of Shiwa-kshar-pachan tablets every 2 hours: then Krimikuthara Rasa every half hour until diarrhœa stops. If diarrhœa does not stop after 8 doses of Krimikuthara Rasa, give Arkadi or Dadimivati Gutika with Arka Churna every two hours until relief.

*LOCALLY.*—Mustard plaster or linseed poultice should be applied over the pit of the stomach to stop vomitting and over the loins to induce the flow of urine.

Cramps and cold are best relieved by friction with the hand or by mustard poultice. In collapse, the patient should be kept warm and the freest ventilation must be secured.

If the breathing is difficult, a mustard poultice should be applied over the chest. Thirst may be quenched by solution of soda water tablet or whey.

*DIET.*—Whey. Great care should be exercised with regard to diet during convalescence; no solid food whatever to be given, until stools are of a natural color. Agni Tundi Guti after meals and Sudarshan Churna in the morning. Rice and whey in diet.

## CHOLERA INFANTUM. *VISHOOCHIKA (Balanani)*

Rest in bed. Stop all food for a time, and give abundance of boiled barley water or whey. Dadimivati pills every 3 hours. If diarrhœa does not stop after 3 doses of Dadimivati pills, give Krimikuthara Rasa in small doses every 2 hours. During convalescence, Samshamani pills 3 times daily and dill water in the morning.

*LOCALLY*--A mustard poultice guarded by muslin should be applied over the abdomen. The extremities should be frequently rubbed with ginger or mustard.

---

## CHYLURIA. *PISTHA MEHA.* S. Ni. Ch. 6. Ch. Chi. Ch.5

This term is applied to a milky condition of the urine.

Vidanga-Tandula Churna *prayoga* (treatment) with Haridradi Quath or Guduchyadi Quath for a fortnight or a month.

After such continued treatment (*prayoga*), Dashanga Abhraka Gutika or Mandura Loha Gutika after meals and Chandraprabha Gutika in the morning should be given for some time; Kapittha leaves powder with honey taken daily for a month or so gives good results.

---

## CIRRHOSIS OF THE LIVER. *YAKRIT-DALYUDAR.* S. Ni. Ch. 7.

*SYMPTOMS.*—The liver becomes atrophied or smaller than natural; the patient becomes despondent and debilitated. The stools which may be loose or the reverse, are generally clay coloured. Sometimes the person becomes jaundiced. Discharge of blood from the bowels and bleeding from the nose are also liable to occur. Regulate diet. Insist on avoidance of stimulants.

*INTERNALLY.*—Eliyakadi Gutika at night and Samudraka Virechan Churna in the morning. If drastic purgative is necessary, give Naracha Rasa. For other treatment, see Hepatitis. Arjuna Twak Quath may be given as heart tonic.

*LOCALLY.*—A blister on the part.

---

## COLIC. *SHOOLA*. S. U. ch. 42.

*RENAL*—Hot Bath. Fomentations with poppy head water. Application of Datura leaves on the part (see Calculi).

*HEPATIC*—Internally—Jatiphaladi Churna Kanaka Sundara Rasa, or Dadimivati Gutika may be given as anodyne, if there is severe pain.

*EXTERNALLY*—Parvativilas Taila or Visha Garbha Taila to be applied on the part; or if necessary, leeches may be applied to liver.

*INTESTINAL*—Recurrent colic may be due to lead poisoning or local disease, *e.g.* gastric ulcer.

*CAREFUL DIET*—Hot water to drink. If stomach is full, and there is need of an emetic give Madanadi Vaman Churna. If bowels are costive, Samudraka Virechana Churna with Hingu Ashtak Churna or Shiwakshar-pachan tikdi. If after two doses of the above medicines given every hour, relief is not obtained, then give Eliyakadi Gutika, with Dadimivati Gutika in small doses followed by Samudraka Virechan Churna after one hour. In severe colic, Shankhvati tikdi may be given for immediate relief.

*EXTERNALLY*—Hot fomentations are useful.

---

## CONJUNCTIVITIS. *ABHISHYANDA*. S U. Ch. 6.

Hot or cold compresses according to the feeling of the patient. Blister behind the ear will relieve inflammation of conjunctivitis on the eye in severe cases. If there is persistent pain, a leech or two may be applied to each temple. Bidalaka Lepa Churna or Rasanjana may be applied to the outside of the eye. In the early stage, two drops of castor oil under the lids. will relieve pain. Latterly lotion of Tuttha tikdi 1 in 4oz. of water or lotion of Shankhadivati tikdi 1 in 1oz. water or lotion of Tankanamla tikdi 1 in 1oz. water is useful.

*INTERNALLY*—Samudraka Virechana Churna as a purgative may be given in the beginning; then Trifala Churna or Trifala Ghrita with milk daily.

---

## CONSTIPATION. *ANAHA.* S. U. Ch. 56. Ch. u. h. 18.

(See Diet tables and general directions).

Insist on regular habit; abdominal massage, morning cold bath and exercise. A glass of cold or hot water taken every morning on rising is often beneficial.

*INTERNALLY*—Purgatives, *e.g.* Shiva-Kshar-Pachan, Abhayadi Modak tikdi, Swadishta Virechana Churna or tikdi, or Samudraka Virechana Churna should be taken.

Use an Enema syringe occasionally.

---

## CONVULSIONS *AKSHEPAK.* S. Ni. Ch. 1. Ch. Su. Ch. 20 (Infantile.)

Treat the exciting cause: *e.g.*, teething, gastro-intestinal disturbance, worms, constipation, onset of acute disease, whooping cough, injuries.

Fresh air should be admitted; the face should be fanned and sprinkled with cold water; the backs should be briskly rubbed; hot baths to the feet. If convulsions occur after a full meal, vomiting should be excited, with hot water or feather (or finger). Castor oil may be given to open the bowels. As calmative, Lakshmi Narayan Rasa may be given in small doses. If the child cannot swallow, castor oil enema may be given

---

## CONVULSIONS PUERPERAL.

Find and remove the cause, Look after the diet. Give as purgative Trivritadi or Samudraka Virechana Churna in the beginning; if drastic purgative be necessary prescribe Naracha Rasa.

As calmative, give Akarkarbhadi Gutika. Hot applications to the feet and cold application to the head.

Examine urine for Albumen (see examination of urine).

Consult expert on women diseases.

## CORNS. *KADAR.* S Ni Ch. 13.

*LOCALLY*—Well fitting boots.

Soak the corn in hot water. and afterwards scratch: if inflamed, rest and poultice should be insisted on.

If the above measures do not succeed, the corns must be burnt with Tuttha tikdi.

## COUGH. *KASA.* S. U Ch. 52. Ch. Chi. Ch 22.

Treat any cause of irritation in the ear, in the larynx, trachea, bronchi, lung, pleura or stomach. In violent paroxysmal cough, think of foreign body in larynx and whooping cough.

*INTERNALLY*—Agnirasa with Arkachurna in the beginning. Lavangadi, Marichyadi, and Kanthya tikdis are beneficial, if allowed to dissolve slowly in the mouth. Confections such as Kantakari-Avaleha, Pippalyadi-leha, Harde-Avaleha or Vasa-Avaleha are useful.

If there is hœmoptysis, give Vasaraga or Vasaleha. For spasmodic cough Krimi Kuthar Rasa is useful.

For painful spasmodic or troublesome cough give Jatiphaladi churna or Akarkarbhadi gutika at bedtime and Agnirasa with Arkachurna in the morning.

*DIET*—Chiefly of milk.

## CORYZA (Catarrh.) *PRATISHYAYA.* S. U. Ch. 24. Ch. Chi. Ch. 26.

Avoid cold temperature, and currents of cold air.

If frequently catching cold, carefully examine nose for enlarged turbinate bones or sensitive spots; throat for enlarged tonsils and chest. Hot baths, and low diet. Feet in hot mustard and water. Hot fomentations to temples. Give Swadishta Virechana Churna or tikdi or Samudraka Virechana Churna in the beginning: then Arka Churna, Lavangadi Churna, or Arkadi tikdi may be given every three hours, or Arkadi tikadi, with Lavangadi Churna in Shunthi Quath in severe cases. Yashtyadi tikdi or Vyoshadi tikadi to be kept in the mouth and allowed to be slowly dissolved,

Quinine sulplate is given by Doctors.

*LOCALLY*—Pinasatamaku Churna to be snuffed. Kasisadi Ghrita to be applied to the nostrils.

For chronic cases, Agnitundi Rasa with Mandurloha gutika or Tonic pills after meals.

## CROUP. *SWARAGHNA.* S. Ni. Ch. 16, Ch. Chi. Ch. 22,

*SYMPTOMS*—In most instances, for some days there is feverishness, accompanied by sneezing, watering of the eyes, and dry cough. The child is probably cross and irritable, and the voice perhaps husky and hoarse. After such premonitory symptoms or without them, the child suddenly awakes with an appearance of suffocation: and with a hoarse ringing cough. The sound of this cough resembles either the crowing of a cock or the bark of a dog, and has a ringing metallic tone. If the disease progresses, tubes or flakes of a whitish membranous substance appear. The efforts to bring up such material are very great; the countenance is flushed, sometimes almost livid, and the body is covered with perspiration, the hands are clenched; the arms thrown about, the eyes project. The pulse is quick, and hard; the skin is burning and thirst is great. The little patient frequently carries the hand to the throat, as if to remove some obstruction.

Treat Catarrh if present. Protect from cold.

*INTERNALLY*—Agnirasa at first, then Arkachurna or Madanadi Vamana churna as an emetic, if necessary. The patient should be given some hot tea or Shunthi Quath, and be covered immediately.

The child should be kept in a warm bath for about eight minutes, being then well and quickly dried and wrapped in blankets.

If Madanadi Vamana Churna gives relief, it may be repeated in about one hour.

The room should be kept warm (see Pneumonia).

If the child is strong and robust, leeches should also be applied over the upper part of the breast bone.

*Diet*—Nutritious.

---

## CYSTITIS. (Inflammation of the bladder) *MUTROUKASAD.* S. U. Ch. 58.

*SYMPTOMS*—Shivering often occurs at first, followed by mental depression, fever, thirst and pain, with tenderness on pressure over the bladder. Pressure in the fork between the legs is also very painful, where there is generally a sense of weight or burning The urine is voided frequently and in small quantities, often with great straining followed by aggravation of the pain and burning. The urine also contains a mucous deposit and sometimes blood.

Rest in bed. Simple diet. Abundant barley water and milk to drink

Treat the cause· *e.g.*, gonorrhœa, stricture, enlarged prostate, calculi, gout, &c.,

Samudraka Virechana Churna in the beginning as a purgative ; then Gokshuradi Avaleha, or Chandraprabha Gutika, with Chandanadi Churna or Garmini tikadi three times a day.

If the pain is severe, Yavakshar with Arkadi tikadi or Jatiphaladi Churna.

*LOCALLY*—Wash bladder out with warm solution of (boric acid) Tankanamla tikadi.

Enema of warm water may be given with benefit.

## DEAFNESS. *BADHIRYA.* S. U. Ch. 20 Ch. Su. Ch. 20.

Seek and treat cause.

If from nervous debility, Pravala Bhasma with Rasayana Churna or Chyavanprasha Avaleha in the morning and Saptamrit Churna with Agnitundi after meals.

If from cold, syringe with warm water, and treat catarrh.

If from enlarged tonsils (see Tonsilitis).

*LOCALLY*—Generally mustard poultice behind the ears. Irimedadi taila dropped in the ear does relief.

## DEBILITY. *KSHINA-ROGA.* Ch. Chi. Ch. 16

Treat dyspepsia if present.

If premonitory to phthisis try to treat it.

If there is mental cause remove it.

Fresh air, rest, change of air, cold or tepid morning bath, with skin friction. If the patient's age be below 40 years, regular and nutritious food with regular exercise will produce beneficial effects.

*INTERNALLY*—Samshamani Gutika, Ashwagandhadi Churna, or Rasayana Churna, with Chyavanaprasha Avaleha or Abhayamalaki Avaleha morning and evening; and Agnitundi Rasa with Manduraloha Gutika or Loha Guggula Gutika after meals.

## DEBILITY (Sexual). *KSHINA SHUKRA KLAIBYA.* S. Sh. Ch. 2. Ch. Chi. Ch. 30.

Attend to the general health, and to the local conditions.

If from exhaustion, as usual, command rest and give Samshamani Gutika, with Ashwa Gandhadi

Churna, Rasayana Churna, Eladi Guti, Shatavaryadi Churna or Musalyadi Churna morning and evening; and Narsinha Churna or Manduraloha Gutika with Agnitundi Rasa after meals. If there is sluggish mentality, add Jatiphaladi Churna at night to the above treatment. Tonic pills if continuously taken for a long time, shows marked benefit.

*DIET*—Nutritious. Milk with Chyavanaprasha Avaleha or Abhayamalaki Avaleha.

Mental rest and sexual abstinence are of very great importance.

---

## DENGUE.

Usually the first symptoms of Dengue, are headache, restlessness, chilliness, debility, pains in the back, limbs, joints and eyeballs, of a very severe character, with more or less feverishness, and often irritability of the stomach. But Dengue sometimes commences with a sudden pain in some joint. Shortly afterwards, an eruption of a red or scarlet character appears on the face, chest, palms and elsewhere, lasting about 48 hours.

Isolate patient. Keep in bed.

Samudraka Virechana churna in the beginning to open the bowels: then if the fever is high, Tripura Bhairava Rasa with parpat quath.

For insomnia and pain of limbs, Jatiphaladi churna or Arkadi tikadi should be used.

Kiratadi quath to be always given during the illness.

Give Swadishta Virechana Churna or Samudraka Virechana churna in small doses to children.

*EXTERNALLY*—Apply Vishagarbha Taila on painful parts, and wrap painful joints in cotton wool.

---

## DIABETES, INSIPIDUS. *UDAKMEHA*. S. Ni Ch. 6. Ch. Chi. Ch. 6

In this disease, very large quantities of urine are passed, but without sugar. (See examination of urine).

Mootrasangrahana quath with Nimbadi quath every morning and evening and Mandurvatak tikdi or Navayasa tikdi after meals.

Akarkarbhadi Gutika, Kanaksunder Rasa or Jatiphaladi Churna in small doses, gives good results.

*DIET*—Dry.

---

## DIABETES MELLITUS. *MADHU MEHA.*

S. Ni. Ch. 6.
Ch. Chi. Ch. 6.

(See diet tables and General Directions).

The treatment of Diabates is more by appropriate diet than by medicines. Samudraka Virechana as a purgative every second or third day.

Then Madhumeha pills No. I, or Salsaradiavaleha, Navayasa tikdi, or Dashang Abhraka Gutika with Agnitundi Rasa after meals for first week; and Madhumeha pills No. II, or Salsaradiavaleha, Navayasa tikdi or Dashang Abhraka Guti, with Dadimivati Gutika after meals for second week. In this way, these medicines should be prescribed alternately for a long time. Swarjikakshar should be given every morning, and Samshamani pills, if necessary.

---

## DIARRHŒA. *ATISAR.*

S. U. Ch. 40.
Ch. Chi. Ch. 10.

See Diet Tables and General Directions.

For irritative diarrhœa, seek cause, which may be one of the following:—Indigestion, worms, retained lumps of faecal matter, overflow of bile: and treat accordingly.

*INTERNALLY*—Castor oil or Shivakshara Pachan; for children, castor oil is best. If there is much griping or nausea, apply a mustard poultice over the bowels.

Diarrhœa resulting from vicissitudes of temperature or mental worry, should not be treated by purgatives; but by stomachic tonic as Pippaliadi churna. If such diarrhœa does not subside spontaneously or by stomachic tonics, Patoladi Yoga quath with Dadimivati Gutika will stop it.

Dysentery sometimes results from this kind of diarrhœa (see Dysentery). In such cases, change of climate is necessary.

---

## DIARRHŒA, CHRONIC. *PAKWA-ATISAR.* S. U. Ch. 40. Ch. Chi. Ch. 10.

Find cause. Examine rectum.

Shriraga Avaleha in the beginning ; if it does not produce good results, add Dadimivati Guti or give Arkadi tikdi with Gangadhar churna.

*DIET*—Whey and rice are the best. If rice do not agree, give only whey.

---

## DIARRHŒA INFANTILE. *BALROGA-ATISAR.*

Sudden diarrhœa with copious greenish watery stools, and great depression should be treated as Cholera. (See Cholera).

*INTERNALLY*—Castor oil in the beginning. then Samshamani guti with Shringiadi churna. If these do not produce any good effects, give Shriraga avaleha, and if even this fails to check the disease, use Dadimivati gutika.

In all cases of Diarrhœa in children, flannel round the bowels is advisable.

If the child is teething, the diarrhœa should not be checked suddenly.

---

## DIPHTHERIA. *KANTH-ROHINI* S. Ni. Ch. 16. Ch. Su. Ch. 18.

The nurse and patient should be isolated from the rest of the family.

*SYMPTOMS*—Ordinarily, the first symptoms are great depression, chilliness, nausea and occasionally diarrhœa. Then the throat begins to feel stiff or tender, with some difficulty of swallowing. At first accompanying the sore throat, there is merely redness of the parts; but in a variable time, characteristic exudation appears, accompanied by badly smelling breath. This may commence at any spot, where the redness has appeared; and generally does so on the tonsils, uvula, soft palate, or on the back of the throat.

At first only small whitish specks may be observed, which speedily extend, and meet, so as to form large patches or to cover the whole surface. The exhudation may spread over the mouth to the lips; it may penetrate the nose; or it may pass into the windpipe occasioning much pain and difficulty of breathing. When the disease has fully formed, there is always hoarse or husky cough, great difficulty in swallowing and fever.

Complete quiet and rest should be observed. The patient's strength must be stored from the first by liberal diet and tonic pills. The patient should be protected from cold and the bowels kept open by Samudraka Virechan churna.

Dry or wet fomentations should be applied to the throat; gargle with solution of Surashtraja tikdi (1 tablet in 4 oz. of water)) or with Shvetadi taila, is beneficial. Kanthya tablets should be sucked. In severe cases, the patient should inhale the steam from hot water, three or four times daily, and strong solution of Surastraja or of Kasis tikdi should be applied to the part every two hours. If food cannot be swallowed by mouth, feeding with nasal or stomach tube is practised by doctors.

---

## DROPSY. *SHOAF* *SHWAYATHU*.

S. Chi Ch. 23.
Ch. Chi. Ch. 17

*GENERAL DIRECTIONS*—Rest. The affected part should be kept raised.

The main point is to remove accumulated fluid by purgatives and diuretics, while the patient's strength should be sustained.

*DIET*—Milk; do not give other fluids except milk.

Treat the cause: Anæmic, hepatic, cardiac, renal.

*ANÆMIC*—Symptoms. Dropsy from Anæmia is rarely extensive and is usually confined to the feet and ankles; fever is probably the premonitory symptom; and the face appears anæmic.

*TREATMENT*—Trikatuadi gutika or Shotha Hara Loha gutika and Arogyavardhani Rasa with Sharapunkha quath or Sudarshana Churna thrice daily.

Daily or alternately, give Samudraka Virechana Churna for constipation.

*DIET*—Milk and rice.

*HEPATIC*—First affects the belly which swells and may be felt to contain fluid.

Eliyakadi Gutika at night, and then Samudraka Virechan Churna in the morning and Arogyavardhani Rasa with Sharpunkha quath. Punarnava quath or Punarnavadi quath, twice a day.

*DIET*—Milk (See Ascites).

*RENAL*—Begins generally in the loose structure of the eyelids and privates, the feet and legs quickly becoming affected. Arogyavardhani Rasa with Punarnava quath in the morning and Chandraprabha gutika or Gokshuradi gutika thrice daily with the same quaths. Samudraka Virechana Churna may be given in the case of constipated bowels. If acute nephritis is the cause, instead of the above medicines, hot fomentations should be applied on the loins.

*CARDIAC*—Commences in the legs and arms often at the same time and gradually involves the whole body. (See Heart-disease).

---

## DYSENTERY *PRAVAHIKA* Ch. Chi. Ch. 10. S. U. Ch. 40.

Rest in bed. Careful diet, *e.g.*, whey and rice. Hot fomentations over the pit of the stomach.

*INTERNALLY*—Castor oil, once in a large dose or twice or thrice in small doses: then Indrayava Churna or Shiva Churna with sugar or Lodhradi Churna, Shriraga avaleha, or Arka Churna or Kutajavaleh, should be given three times a day.

For more acute forms of dysentery Arkadi tikdi or Dadimivati with Shriraga avaleha three times a day, after castor oil. If there is fever, give Samshamani pills with Parpat quath.

## DYSENTERY Chronic. *PRAVAHIKA.* S. U. Ch. 40. Ch. Chi. Ch. 10

Repeated applications of mustard poultices over the tender parts of the bowels. A flannel belt should be worn round the bowels.

*INTERNALLY*—Castor oil for constipation and Arkadi tikdi or Devkusumadi rasa with Shriraga avaleha or Dadimatwak quath, when the bowels are loose.

Treat piles if present.

Guduchyadi quath in the morning for dyspepsia.

*DIET*—Whey only; or hot milk frequently in small quantities.

## DYSENTERY IN CHILDREN.

Perfect cleanliness.

Castor oil twice or thrice a day, and Arkaditikdi at night.

After two days, instead of castor oil
to a child up to 6 months old ¼ gr. Arka Churna
" " " 12 months old 1 gr. " "
" " " 2 years old 2 gr. " "
should be given three times a day and Arkadi tikdi at night. Samshamani guti for a few days after cure.

## DYSMENORRHŒA. *ARTAV-DOSH-KRATCHHARAJASKA.*

S. ·ha. . h. 2. Ch. Chi. Ch. 30.

Avoid exposure to damp or chill or excitement of any kind for three or four days previous to the expected period. Take care against constipation.

*REST*—Hot mustard hip baths. After baths, flannels wrung out of hot water should be applied over the lower part of the bowels and privates.

*INTERNALLY*—Eliyadi gutika to be commenced three days previous to the expected period: Krimikuthar Rasa as an anodyne, when pain is severe. If the discharge continues for longer period, give Karpasmul quath.

During intervals Kasisadi gutika and Agnitundi rasa after meals.

Ascertain if there is any mechanical obstruction.

---

## DYSPEPSIA. *AGNIMANDYA.* Ch. Chi.Ch. 19 Ma. Ni.

(See diet tables and general directions)

For an acute attack of indigestion, only hot water or sodawater tablet may be given. Madanadi Vaman Churna if an emetic seems necessary.

*LOCALLY*—Fomentations with hot water or mustard poultice.

For chronic dyspepsia, Hinguashtak Churna, Vadavanal Churna, Vaishvanar Churna, or Bhaskar Lavan Churna fifteen minutes before meals; Agnitundi rasa after meals; and Kiratadi quath, Bhunimbadi churna, Sudarshana churna or Arogyavardhani rasa every morning and evening.

---

## DYSURIA. *MUTRAKRICHHA.* S. U. Ch. 59.

There is difficulty in discharging the urine attended with pain and a sensation of heat.

*TREAT CYSTITIS*—Give cold bath and diuretic and demulcent drugs, *e.g.* Mutravirechan quath, Virtarvadigana quath, Brahatyadigana quath, Eladi churna, Gokshurakadiavaleha, Gokshuradi gutika, Chandraprabha gutika. Barley water, water with Isapgula, Gokshuraka or Balabija should be taken in abundance.

*DIET*—Abundant milk.

## EAR-ACHE. *KARNASHOOLA.* S. U. Ch. 21. Ch. Chi. Ch. 26

Examine carefully ear, mouth, teeth, throat and nose. Wash mouth, and gargle throat frequently with hot water.

*LOCALLY*—Hot fomentations (with water or poppy head water). Irrigation with hot saline solution. Blister or leeches behind ear. Vishagarbha taila or Paravativilas taila should be dropped in the ear.

*INTERNALLY*—Jatifaladi Churna as anodyne and castor oil or Samudraka Virechan churna as a mild purgative. Samshamani guti may be given with advantage.

---

## EAR (Inflammation of the) *KARNASHOATH.* S, U. Ch. 20

Apply leeches behind the ear.

Fresh leeches after six hours if necessary.

Fomentations of poppy water or hot water.

Vishagarbha taila or Parvativilas taila should be dropped in the ear.

*INTERNALLY*—Samudraka Virechan churna or Ashwa Kanchuki gutika as purgative for adults, and castor oil for children. Syringe should not be used except to clear away discharge.

### Chronic Inflammation—

Perfect cleanliness.

The ear should be gently syringed daily with warm lotion of Jantughna and Grahi tikdi (1 in 10 oz. of water) and dried carefully.

Blister behind the ear. Protection of the ear by cotton wool loosely placed in the orifice.

Insist on avoidance of cold or draught.

*INTERNALLY*—Saptamrit churna and Agnitundi rasa or tonic pills after meals.

Attend to general health.

## ECZEMA. *KITIBH.* S. Ni. Ch. 5. Ch. Chi. Ch. 7.

Protect against all irritation: heat, sun, discharges. Wash little, use milk and water, or oat meal water or almond oil on soft linen. Keep the folds of the skin apart. Attend to the diet and digestion and regulate bowels.

Examine urine for sugar and albumen.

*LOCALLY*—Poultices if there is swelling or pain. Crusts may be removed by poultices: then Dadrughna malam or Turushkadi malam should be applied in the daytime; and Rasa Karpuradi taila should be vigorously rubbed over the part at night.

*INTERNALLY*—Debility, anæmia, constipation, fever, must be cured as directed under those headings.

Samshamani guti should be always given.

The treatment should be continued for a long time.

---

## ELEPHANTIASIS. *SHLIPAD.* Ch. Chi. Ch. 17 S. Ni. Ch. 11.

Avoidance of all impure drinking is imperative. Care must be taken to keep the skin folds clean.

Application of a bandage first soaked in a solution containing 5 grs. of Kasis tikdi in 1 oz. of warm water. If sores form between the toes, Jasata Pushpa should be dusted over the part. An elastic bandage or stocking will give ease by supporting the tissues of the limb.

*INTERNALLY*—castor oil for one month and Trifala Gugula gutika or Kaishor Gugula gutika with Manjishtadi quath twice daily till relief.

*DIET*—milk and rice.

---

## EMISSIONS (Nocturnal).

Keep the bowels regular: treat worms if present: avoid stimulants: avoid all fluids for two hours before bed time. The bladder to be emptied after first deep sleep. Avoid lying on the back. Exercise and cold hip bath at night.

Samudraka Virechan churna or Shiva churna may be given at first to remove constipation, if necessary; then Saptamrit churna or Rasayan churna with honey twice a day. If discharge is too often, give Krimikuthar rasa. For debility, Agnitundi rasa with Manduraloha guti; Narsinha churna or tonic pills after meals.

---

## EPILEPSY. *APASMAR.* Ch. Chi. Ch. 15. S. U. Ch. 61.

Treat any possible cause of irritation, *e.g.* brain-tumour, uterine trouble, intestinal worms, teething, irregularity of monthly flow, indigestion, etc. Maintain the general health with good food, fresh air, and tonics. Prohibit alcohol, tobacco, bad habits, (masterbation), and animal food. Insist on exercise and more milk in diet.

If the stomach is full when warnings are felt Madanadivaman Churna or mustard water, will sometimes stop a fit; if the stomach is not full, draught of cold water.

*DURING THE FIT*—The patient must be prevented injuring himself. Fresh air should be admitted freely and the face should be fanned and freely douched with cold water.

Navasagar and fresh lime mixed freshly, or good tobacco should be inhaled.

*DURING INTERVALS*—Kanaksunder rasa Jatiphaladi churna or Arkadi tikdi with Brahmighrita or Siddharaka ghrita morning and evening and Medhya Rasayan Churna, Chitrak Mooladi Churna, or Amarsundari rasa, may be given after meals.

In Alopathy, during fit, Amil Nitrite is given for inhalation, and during intervals, Potassium Iodide and Potassium Bromide.

---

## EPISTAXIS. *NASARAKTA, RAKTAPITTA, URDHWAGATA.* Ch. Chi. Ch. 25 S. U. Ch. 22.

Examine nose for local cause.

Treat associated conditions, *e.g.*, Bright's disease, (Vrikka-shoath) typhoid fever, new growth.

*DURING ATTACK*—Rest with the head raised ; cold application to back of neck. Warmth to hands and feet.

*LOCALLY*—Plug the bleeding nostril with cotton wool saturated in solution of Surastraja tikdi or of Kasis tikdi. Injection of cold water. For habitual epistaxis, drop Chandanadi taila or almond oil in the nostril.

*INTERNALLY*—Vasaraga with 1 gr. of Kasis tikdi in the morning and Chandraprabha guti in the evening. If there is debility, Chandrakala rasa or Saptamrit churna with Dashasar tikdi after meals. Chyavanprasha avaleh in the morning as nutritious diet.

---

## ERYSIPELAS. *VISARPA.* S. Ni. Ch. 10. Ch. Chi. Ch. 11.

Fresh air without draughts. Perfect cleanliness.

*LOCALLY*—The part affected should be covered with lint soaked in tepid water or with lepa of Manjishthadi churna, Mustadi churna or Dashang lepa churna, over which oiled silk should be laid. The red area must be freely painted with strong solution of Kasis tikadi for two inches beyond the red margin, so that the disease will not spread.

A purgative as castor oil or Samudraka Virechan churna is generally required at first. Then if there is fever, Tripurbhairav rasa or Samshamani guti with Parpat quath. For debility, Mandurloha guti with Agnitundi rasa after meals, and nutritious food.

If the disease is not cured with the above treatment, leeches may be applied or a knife used, and the blood is let out. After operation, for treatment of ulcer, (See Ulcer).

---

## FAINTING. *MOORCHHA.* S. U. Ch. 46. Ch. Su. Ch. 19.

*DURING ATTACK*—Keep the head low ; place the body in a recumbent position. Apply cold water to the face. Allow cold air into the room. Take the person out of doors. Rub the limbs well. A burnt feather should be held smoking under the nose or Navasagar mixed with fresh lime should be given as a smelling salt.

Vidang churna or Shirovirechan churna may be given as sternutatory. If a stimulant is required, Drakshasara should be given.

If fainting continues longer, a mustard poultice may be applied on the chest. Rest will cure the subsequent languor. For the prevention of a fainting fit, lying down at full length without a pillow under the head is necessary. Persons subject to fainting usually require outdoor exercise and they should avoid constipated bowels and should take Samshamani guti with Draksh (grapes) in the morning and Mandurloha guti with Agnitundi rasa after meals.

---

## FEVER. *JWARA.* Ch. Chi. Ch. 3. S. U. Ch. 39.

*DURING HOT STAGE*—Hot tea, Shunthi quath and if the fever is below 104°, steam bath should be given ; but if it rises higher, a wet towel should be placed over the bowels and covered by a blanket. The towel should be changed every 10 or 15 minutes. For vomiting (see Vomiting). For headache, ice or lotion of Shital tikdi on the head.

*MEDICINES DURING ATTACK*—Samudraka Virechan Churna or Ashwakanchuki rasa as purgative, if necessary.

As diaphoretic, Chandraprabha and Parpat quath with Vacha churna or Arkachurna. Ratnagiri rasa, Tribhuvankirti rasa, Tripur Bhairav rasa or Krimikuthar rasa with Parpat quath.

*DURING CONVALESCENCE*-Ashwakanchuki rasa or Samudraka Virechan Churna to clear bowels. As antipyretic, Guduchyadi quath, Saptaparna quath, Mahajwarankusha rasa, Chakri rasa, Kalingakadi quath, Narayan Jvarankusha rasa and Kiratadi quath are useful.

After debility, Sudarshana Churna with Samshamani guti three times a day for a few days.

**FEVER** *SHEET JWAR.* Ch. Chi. Ch. 3. S. U. Ch. 39.
**(Intermittent.)**

*DURING COLD STAGE*—Hot bricks or hot water bottles to the feet, a pan containing hot ashes under the bed.

Hot Shunthi quath or tea.

*DURING HOT STAGE*—Cold application, *e.g.* ice or lotion of Shital tikdi on the head. Wet pack over the bowels.

*INTERNALLY*—Samudrakvirechan churna in small doses in the beginning. If temperature rises high, Tripurbhairav Rasa with Parpat quath or other diaphoretics should be given. When the patient begins to perspire, the body should be covered; and hot tea or Shunthi quath given to drink.

*DURING CONVALESCENCE,*—Samudrak virechan churna or Ashwakanchuki rasa should be given as purgative at first; then Saptaparna quath, Guduchyadi quath, or other antipyretics should be administered. (See Fever).

*Quinine is administered by doctors.*

---

**FEVER** *SUTIKA JWARA.* Ma. Ni.
**(Puerperal.)**

*INTERNALLY*—Samudraka Virechan churna in the beginning. If fever is very high, Ratnagiri rasa with Devdaravadi quath or Dashmul quath should be given; otherwise Samshamani guti with the same quath.

Expert of women diseases should be consulted at once.

---

**FEVER** *PARIVARTI JWAR—* Bhav..
**(Relapsing)** *SANNIPATBHEDA*

*SYMPTOMS*—In this type of fever, the temperature rises more or less rapidly up to a certain point and then remains tolerably stationary for a time and finally defervescence and apparent recovery take place; but this is followed after some days by a relapse—which course of events may be repeated more than once.

*TREATMENT*—Perfect cleanliness. Abundance of liquid and easily digested food, cautiously. At first Samudraka Virechan churna or Ashwakanchi rasa in the beginning as purgative.

*DURING HOT PERIOD*—Chandraprabha gutika with Parpat quath. If there is collapse, Draksharasa or Agnitundi rasa.

*DURING CONVALESCENCE*—Agnitundi rasa for debility: Guduchyadi quath, Chakri rasa or Narayan Jwarankusha as Antipyretic. (See Fever.)

*AFTER FULL RECOVERY*—Manduraloha gutika and Agnitundi rasa after meals and Samshamani guti three times daily for a few days with nutritious food.

*LOCALLY*—Wet packing, cold application on the head, &c., as directed in fever.

---

## FEVER (Remittent.) *JWAR SANTAT*

S. U. Ch. 39. Ch. Chi. Ch. 3.

Symptoms may commence as an intermittent fever; the intermissions becoming less marked, until after a few days, that is the period between the paroxysms shows only a lowering of body temperature, not a return to normal. The symptoms of remittent fever are those of ague without distinct stages. The fever continues frequently for 8 hours, characterized by the pulse becoming quicker, heavy breathing with great restlessness—the temperature being often as early as the evening of the second day as high as 106° Farh, and the pulse varying from 100 to 120.

Typhoid fever being the disease with which remittent fever is most usually confused, the chief distinctive points are given below :—

| *Typhoid.* | *Remittent.* |
|---|---|
| Onset gradual. | Onset sudden. |
| Shivering little marked. | Shivering more marked. |
| Temperature does not rise at first for some days. | Early rise of temperature often on first day. |
| Origin connected with defective conservancy. | Origin connected with exposure to malaria. |

| *Typhoid.* | *Remittent.* |
|---|---|
| Usually diarrhœa from the first, with yellow 'stools' (dull yellow) | Constipation at first, or dark bilious 'stools' (coach-paint yellow). |
| Tenderness and pain of bowels. | Tenderness over the spleen and over the stomach after vomiting |
| Eruption of rose or pink coloured spots. | None. |
| Remission of fever slight and nearly always in the morning. | Daily remissions, generally occurring in the early morning, but also at other times. |
| Jaundice very seldom occurs. | Often occurs. |
| Gastric symptoms, as nausea, hiccough and vomiting, occasional. | Gastric symptoms nearly always present. |

*TREATMENT*—Perfect rest. Give Samudraka Virechan Churna in the morning in the beginning only until the stools are of a healthy yellow colour.

During hot stage, Chandraprabha guti with Kiratadi quath, Saptaparna quath or Gudchyad quath. During remission, quinine should be administered with Chandraprabha, until two days have passed without fever. For vomiting soda-water tablet should be given. Agnitundi rasa for debility.

For treatment of headache and other symptoms, see Fever.

*DIET*—Nutritious.

---

## FEVER- (Typhoid.) *SANNIPAT JWAR* (*Pralapak*). S. U. Ch. 3. Ch. Chi. Ch. 3.

See diet tables and general directions.

*SYMPTOMS*—Stomach derangement as nausea, vomiting, and inability to retain food, may be from the commencement. At length, the pulse becomes quicker and full; the skin hot and dry, and at about the end of the first week, the patient takes to his bed with appetite gone, the tongue coated, and the bowels loose. The fever now shows an increase in the afternoon, and a slight remission towards morning. The diarrhœa continues, the stools are thin, of a yellow colour, and have a characteristic odour. If now the hand is pressed on the right side of the abdomen, the patient's face will express pain and a gurgling may also be felt and heard under the fingers. The abdomen becomes tense and resonant (tympanitic). Between the seventh and twelfth days, the eruption of typhoid fever appears on the chest, abdomen and back, consisting of a few slightly raised rose coloured spots, which disappear temporarily on pressure. In severe cases about the middle of the second week, delirium comes on—at first slight and afterwards more constant, intense and noisy. As the malady increases, the tongue becomes drier, red and glazed, and often cracks in various directions, while dry brown crusts form on the teeth. The lips also crack and bleed. The patient loses flesh and strength rapidly, lies prostrate, and is often unconscious. Dilated pupils, bleeding from the nose, blood passed with stools, urine and stools passed involuntarily, muttering delirium and convulsions, are all unfavourable symptoms.

*TREATMENT*—Perfect cleanliness. The mouth and teeth should be kept clean.

For treatment of vomiting, headache and other symptoms, see Fever.

No solid food should be allowed for six weeks or two months. Only milk should be allowed.

*INTERNALLY*—For fever and as an intestinal antispetic, Ratnagiri rasa with Parpat quath. The diarrhœa at first need seldom be checked. Only Arkachurna in 2 grs. doses should be given night and morning. But if purging is more than 8 or 9 times a day, or if there is bleeding from the bowels, give Panchamrit Parpati rasa. For debility, give Agnitundi rasa; for delirium, Jatiphaladi churna.

## FISSURE OF THE ANUS.

*INTERNALLY*—Swadishta Virechan churna, every day or every other day.

*LOCALLY*—Extreme cleanliness—washing with soap and water, or with solution of Jantughna and Grahi tablet (1 in 10 oz. of water) or with solution of Surastraja tablet.

Rasanjana, Jatyadi malam or Kashisadi malam should be applied in ulcer.

If the fissure is deep or large, rest and surgical operation may be required.

---

## FISTULA ET ANO. *BHAGANDAR.* S. Ni. Ch. 4. Ch. Chi. Ch. 17.

(See Sinus).

The disease requires operation.

After operation, it should be dressed with Chitrakadi taila; Magadhyadi taila, Jatyadi malam or Kashisadi malam.

Ahiphenadi malam is good for application as an anodyne.

*INTERNALLY*—Vidangady-avaleha, Swyambhoova Gugula gutika, Kishor Gugula gutika or Devakusumadi rasa with Manjishthadi quath thrice daily.

---

## GIDDINESS. *BHRAMA.* Ch. Su. Ch. 20. ? a. Ni.

Treat cause, *e.g.*, debility, disordered stomach, indigestion, gout, heart disease, &c. Giddiness is also premonitory of epilepsy, apoplexy, or fainting.

(For treatment see those diseases).

Rest in the horizontal position and castor oil syringe will give temporary relief. For permanent relief, Eliyakadi gutika at night and Samudraka Virechan churna next morning for two or three days: then Samshamani pills with Shunthi quath in the morning and Manduraloha gutika with Agnitundi rasa after meals. If there is liver complaint, give Arogyavardhani rasa.

*DIET*—Nutritious, *e.g.* milk, Chyavanprash, &c.

---

## GOITRE. *GALGAND.* S. Nl. Ch. 11. Ch. Chi. Ch. 17.

The enlargement of the thyroid gland. The gland lies on either side; the middle line just above the breast bone. The tumour is generally irregularly ovoid, elastic, and free from the pain It sometimes attains a great size, *causing*, by pressing on the windpipe and blood vessels of the part, *difficulty of breathing, difficulty of swallowing, headache and change in the pitch of voice.*

Attend to general health. Change of residence

*INTERNALLY*—Guduchyadi quath.

*LOCALLY*—Fomentations with hot water or poultices. Doshaghna Churna lepa or Manjishthadi Churna lepa should be applied.

Pardadi malam or Rasakurpuradi taila should be freely applied and the neck then exposed to the rays of the sun or to a brisk fire.

If the gland is removed by operation, the ulcer should be washed daily with solution of Jantughna tikdi (1in 20 oz. of water).

*INTERNALLY*—Samudraka Virechan churna in the beginning.

*DIET*—Barley and barley water.

*IN ALOPATHY*—Potassium Iodide is given internally and Red Iodide of Mercury is used externally.

---

## GONORRHŒA. *OUPSARGIK-MEHA.* Bhai.

Avoid exercise, alcohol, tobacco, coffee, cheese, pepper, spices and all stimulating food.

Rest—Suspensory bandage, warm baths, frequent hot fomentations to perinæum; perfect cleanliness, hot hip baths.

*INTERNALLY*—Samudraka Virechan churna in the beginning; then Yavakshara or Chandraprabha guti and Gurmini tikdi or sandal wood oil and cubeb oil, every two hours. If the burning pain is unbearable, Jatiphaladi churna should be given.

*LOCALLY*—Urethra should be syringed with Panchvalkal quath or Mehantak lotion.

Doctors wash with Permanganate of Potash solution.

Drink plenty of water, barley water or linseed water.

Gokshuradi Gugula gutika with Trivritadi quath taken for a long time will prevent the after effects of gonorrhœa, *e.g.* gleet.

---

## GOUT. *VATARAKTA.* S. Ni. Ch. 1. Ch. Chi. Ch. 29.

See diet tables and general directions.

*SYMPTOMS*—A fit of gout is usually preceded by irritability of temper, feverishness and headache; most frequently comes on during the night. There is acute grinding pain in the part—most usually the great toe, abating towards the morning, but leaving the toe red and swollen ; tender and shining. There is also acid perspiration and the urine at first scanty, high coloured and clear, afterwards becomes more copious and deposits a sediment, resembling pounded brick dust. For several nights, the pain may return, although it is usually lessened as the swelling increases. As the pain and swelling subside, the skin of the part peels off in flakes. The disease then disappears perhaps not returning for months. Repeated attacks may lead to ulcers and chalk stones. Gout may occur in the fingers with similar results. In rarer cases, it may suddenly leave the toe and attack the stomach. Gout may also attack other internal organs.

On approach of the attack, the bowels, if confined, should be relieved by Elivakadi guti at night and Samudraka Virechan churna in the morning. Then Chandraprabha gutika with Trivritadi quath, or Kaishor gugula guti, or Amrita gugul guti, with Trivritadi quath mixed with Kshardwaya churna three times daily.

*DURING ATTACK—Internally :* Dadimivati guti or headache cure tablet and Trivritadi quath mixed with Kshardwaya churna should be given.

*LOCALLY*—Vishagarbha taila to be applied on the part ; Tiladi lepa may be applied on the part like poultice.

*AVOID* ice—cold applications to a very inflamed joint.

Raise the part and wrap it up in cotton wool.

Foment the part with hot poppy head water or hot Swarjika lotion (4 drms. in 1 oz. of water).

---

## HEART-BURN. *HRADAYADAH.* S.Su.Ch. 46

Treat dyspepsia.

In the beginning, a full draught of hot water with or followed (after 15 minutes) by Swarjika kshara.

Between the attacks, Shunthyadi tikdi, Hingnadi churna or Shivaksharpachan should be given twice a day and a draught of cold water at night. If the patient is costive, Avipattikara tikadi with Sudarshan churna in the morning and Drakshadı tikdi after meals.

*DIET*—Fruits after meals.

---

## HEMATEMESIS. *PITTAJANYA-CHHARDI–OORDHWAGAT RAKTAPITTA.* S. U. Ch. 45. Ch. Chi. Ch. 4.

The blood vomited from the stomach is almost of black colour, but if the blood is discharged immediately after its escape into the stomach, it may be quite bright. The quantity of blood discharged necessarily varies much and it is generally more or less mixed with food, preceded or accompanied by burning painin the istomach. If the ulcer is large the blood is sufficient to cause alarming faintness.

Treat cause. *e.g.* gastric ulcer, gastric cancer, alcoholism, diseases of liver, spleen and kidney. Treat anæmia and constipation.

The distinction between bleeding from the lungs and bleeding from the stomach :—

| *Hœmoptysis or bleeding from the lungs.* | *Hœmatamesisor bleeding from the stomach.* |
|---|---|
| Usually difficulty of breathing, pain in chest. | Nausea, pain, tenderness at the pit of the stomach |
| Blood coughed up in mouthfuls | Blood vomited profusely |
| Blood frothy | Blood not frothy. |
| Blood of a florid red colour. | Blood generally dark coloured. |
| Blood mixed with saliva. | Blood mixed with food. |
| No blood passed by 'stools' | Blood often passed by 'stool'. |
| Cough and bronchial symptoms | None. |

Avoid stimulants.

When gastric ulcer is the cause, stop food to give absolute rest to the stomach.

Milk should be given frequently in small quantities. If cow's milk is not retained in the stomach. goat or donkey's milk may be given. Barley water may also be tried. Milk mixed with lime water given every two hours in as much quantity as can be taken is the chief treatment.

*TREATMENT*—Dadimivati and Kasis tikdi with Karpasmool quath, three times a day. If milk is not retained at all, nutrient enema of milk with Kasis tikdi and Dadimivati may be given per rectum.

---

## HÆMATURIA, *SHONIT MEHA.* S. Ni. Ch. 6. Ch. Chi. Ch. 6.

Treat the cause, *e.g.* gonorrhœa, calculi, tubercle of the kidney or bladder, nephritis, prostatis, &c. (See examination of urine).

*INTERNALLY*—Give Garmini tikdi or Chandraprabha guti with Trivritadi quath, three times a day.

*LOCALLY*—Hot fomentation or mustard poultice on the loins, if nephritis is the cause. A towel wet with solution of Shital tikdi on the lower part of the bowels.

Barley water, Isapfgul water or Gokshurak water should be given to drink.

---

**HAEMOPTYSIS.** *OORDHWAGATA RAKTAPITTA OORAKSHAT.* S. U. Ch. 41. Ch. Chi. Ch. 16.

Is often a symptom of consumption(see Phthisis)

Frothy bright coloured blood is coughed up; there may be pain and a sensation of bubbling in the chest.

Perfect quiet; rest in bed. Avoid use of voice.

In the beginning, if the patient is strong enough Arkachurna should be given in small doses every one hour. After five or seven doses of Arkachurna if no effect is apparent, then give solution of Kasistikdi or Surastraja tikdi with Dadimivati. Vasaraga or Vasaleha with Trifala Churna or only Vasavaleha are also beneficial.

Milk with Laksharasa has also been found efficacious.

*LOCALLY*—Hot water bag to spine.

*DIET*—Milk. Goat milk is preferable.

Drink cold water, fresh lemon water, lime water or iced acid drink.

---

**HEADACHE.** *SHIRAH-SHOOL.* S. U. Ch. 25. Ch. Chi. Ch. 26.

(See Hemicrania)

For dyspeptic headache, give sodawater tablet every four hours till relieved. If headache is also due to constipation, give Samudraka Virechana churna or Shivakshar pachan as a laxative,

If headache commences shortly after a meal. Madanadi Vaman churna will relieve it.

When the liver or bowels are most in fault, give Eliyakadi guti at night and Samudraka virechan churna in the morning.

For immediate relief, headache cure tablet is best.

## HEART (Diseases of).

**Maintain the general health.**

**Prohibit overwork or fatigue of body or mind.**

**Attend to digestion. Take regular exercise.**

**If dropsy of the legs appear, rest in bed is essential.**

**For pain, give rest, Drakshasava or Agnitundi guti internally; and locally apply mustard poultices to the heart.**

**For Dropsy: Trivritadi quath, or Samudrak Virechan churna should be given to produce watery stools. Kakubhadi churna or Arjun quath may be given as heart tonic.**

---

## HEMICRANIA. *ARDHAVBHEDAK.* S. U. Ch. 25.

**Always seek cause for chronic or oft-recurring headache; brain tumour, nasal obstruction, decayed teeth, &c.**

**Regulate the diet. Treat constipation. Prohibit overwork. Insist on rest in bed during attack.**

***INTERNALLY*—In the interval, Samudrak Virechan churna in the beginning; then as tonic, tonic pills, or Saptamrit churna with Pathyadi quath.**

**During attack, prescribe headache cure tablet or Lakshminarayan guti.**

---

## HEMIPLEGIA. *PAKSHAGHAT-PAKSHVADHA.* Ch. Su. Ch. 20 S. Ni. Ch. 1.

***INTERNALLY*—Vatarirasa or Ekangvira rasa with Maha Yograj gugulla guti or Swayambhoo gugula guti and Rasanadi quath three times a day.**

***LOCALLY*—Apply Vishagarbha taila on the part.**

***DIET*—Nutritious.**

## HEPATITIS. *YAKRIT-DALYUDAR.* Ch. Chi. Ch. 18. S. Ni. Ch. 7.

*INTERNALLY*—Eliyakadi guti in the morning followed by Samudraka virechan churna after three hours; if the bowels are costive, and there is no dysenteric complication, the above medicines should be administered every other day. Navsagar with Arogyavardhani should be given three times daily, and Sharpunkha quath, Rohitak quath or Nimbadi quath twice daily.

If pain continues, a blister should be applied over the part. Internally, tonic pills should be given after meals.(See Anaemia).

*DIET*—Milk and fruits.

If there is abscess of liver, operation is imperative.

---

## HERNIA. *ANTRA VRIDHHI.* S. Ni. Ch. 12.

*DURING ATTACK*—Application of solution of Shital tikdi (or ice). Compression by hand.

The foot of bed being raised two or three feet from the floor, the patient should be let alone for two or three hours. Sometimes an operation is necessary.

*DURING CONVALESCENCE*—Bowels should be kept open by castor oil or by Samudrak virechan churna when necessary and Kindaru churna with Kirat churna or Kuberaksh churna and Sindhav, daily.

For infantile hernia, the same medicines in small doses.

A hernia bandage should be worn.

*DIET*—Fluid and unconstipative.

---

## HERPES ZOSTER. *KAKSHA.* S. Ni. Ch. 18. Ch. Chi. Ch. 17.

In this form of Herpes, a line of vesicles rises reaching from the spine, round the lower part of the chest, or abdomen, to the middle line usually on one side.

Regulate diet; avoid scratching. Keep the bowels open by Samudrak Virechan churna. If there is fever, Tripurbhairav rasa or Chandraprabha guti and Samshamani guti with Parpat quath should be given. Tonic pills as general tonic.

*LOCALLY*—Lotion of Surashtraja tikdi (1 tablet in 4 oz. of water) should be applied. If the pain is severe, Jantughna and Grahi lotion (1 tablet in 10 oz. of water) or hot poppy water should be applied.

## HICCOUGH. *HIKKA* · U. Ch. 50. Ch. Chi. Ch. 21.

Treat Dyspepsia, correct diet, and give dry meals.

Hold the breath, drink hot water, sneeze: sip cold water. Use tight belt over the abdomen.

*TREATMENT*—Shunthyadi tikdi or Hingnadi churna will probably give relief. Madanadi Vaman churna as an emetic, if stomach is full. Smoke from burnt peacock feathers applied to the nostrils, will stop hiccough. Harde-avaleha is also beneficial.

## HOARSENESS-LARYNGITIS. *SWAR-BHEDA.* S. U. Ch. 53. Ch. Chi. Ch. 26.

When the malady presents as simple hoarseness avoid cold, especially at night. Wrap flannel round the throat. Prohibit talking. When the disease is severe, leeches should be applied to the chest. The feet should be kept in mustard water at night. If the patient be a child, it should be put to bed. Steam from hot water should be frequently inhaled. Hot moist sponges applied to the throat. The air should be rendered moist by steam from a kettle of boiling water.

Medhya Rasayan churna or Arkachurna and Vasaraga to adults.

To the child patient in severe hoarseness, Chandraprabha guti with Tripurbhairav rasa in small doses and Parpat quath for fever and Arkadi tikdi every four hours to relieve pain. If the patient is a strong robust person, Madanadi Vamna churna may at first be given as an emetic and then Devkusumadi rasa instead of Arkadi tikdi.

If the bowels are costive, laxative pills at night and Samudraka Virechan churna in the morning.

Yashthyadi tikdi may be given to suck in all cases.

---

## HYDROPHOBIA. *JALTRAS.* S. Ka. Ch. 6.

The patient should, as soon as possible, be sent, with the certificate of a qualified medical practitioner, to the Kasauli Pasteur Institute, for Pasteur serum treatment.

As immediate measures, a tight bandage over the bite, which must be washed with Panchvalkal quath and caustic-ed with Rasakarpura or Dalchikna (Doctors usually wash with Permanganate of Potash solution and then caustic with pure nitrate of silver) or burnt with a red hot knife blade.

Always avoid a gloomy view of the case. Cheer up the sufferer as much as possible. Give Jatiphaladi churna or Kanaksunder rasa to calm the excitement.

---

## HYSTERIA. *APTANTRAK.* S. Ni. Ch. 1.

Mental weakness and sexual desire are often the causes of hysteria.

Attend to general health.

*DURING ATTACK*—Massage: cold water to the chest and head; snuff to be inhaled, a fan should be used (Eau de cologne is sprinkled on the face); smoke from burnt feathers applied to the nostrils.

*INTERNALLY*—Krimikuthar rasa or Dwiruttar Hinguadi churna every hour for recurring fits. Ordinarily, Amarsundarivati or Yograj guti with Samshamani guti twice a day for some time. Good food, good exercise, employment for the mind: attention to the bowels and cold baths are necessary. Agnitundi rasa after meals, for debility. If the monthly flow is deficient or irregular, it must be treated.

## INCONTINENCE OF URINE. *HASTI-MEHA.* S. Ni. Ch. 6. Ch. Chi. Ch. 6.

In adults, this disease is often a sign of retention, indicating residual urine, as in enlarged prostrate or other long standing urethral obstruction and in certain nervous diseases.

In children, it may be due to general ill health or to thread worms, constipation, phimosis, enlarged tonsils, abnormal urine; or irritation of the bladder (as from stone).

*TREATMENT FOR ADULTS*—Give Chandraprabha guti or Gokshuradi guti in the morning; Agnitundi rasa after meals, and Kanaksunder rasa or Akarkarbhadi guti at night. Wake the child up in the night to micturate. Prohibit drinking water in the evening. Treat cause. Samshamani guti with Shringyadi churna in the morning and Mandurvatak tikdi after meals.

## INDIGESTION. *AJIRNA.* S. Su. Ch. 45.

Seek the cause and treat it. Give Shivaksharpachan or Samudraka Virechan churna for indigestion caused by overeating. If with constipation, give Abhayadi Modak tikdi, Trivritadi churna or Laxative pills. Also hot water and Swarjika-kshar and Hingu-ashtak churna for acid indigestion with heart burn. Give Shankhavati tikdi, Sanjivni guti, Kravyad or Krimikuthar rasa if there is diarrhœa, tympanitis or colic.

Agnitundi rasa with Sudarshan Churna to give tone to the stomach. (See Anorexia, constipation, cholera, acidity, dyspepsia, heart-burn, &c.)

## INFLUENZA. *DUSHTA PRATISHYAYA.* S. U. Ch. 24.

This is a severe epidemic catarrh. The symptoms of influenza are first, those of a very bad cold (catarrh) to which are added, a sudden early and extraordinary loss of strength, great depression of spirits, restlessness and anxiety with fever. There is usually cough ; and there is always danger of bronchitis or inflammation of the lungs. The very young and the very old bear influenza less favourably.

The patient should be placed in bed in a cool, well-ventilated room, but free from draughts. In the beginning, Samudrak Virechan churna should be given to subdue feverishness and open bowels ; then Samshamani guti with Sudarshan churna or Tripurbhairav rasa with Parpat quath, if the temperature is more than 103°.

For cough, Arkachurna with Vasaraga. Drak-sharasa may be given for debility.

After two or three days, nutritious diet such as milk and rice should be given. If bronchitis, pneumonia or rheumatism occur, the treatment for those affections should be pursued.

---

## INSOMNIA. *ASWAPNA-NIDRANASH*,

S. U. Ch. 61.
Ch. Su. Ch. 20.

Remove the cause when possible, *e.g.*, anæmia, latent gout, dyspepsia, mental anxiety, alcohol. tobacco, strong tea or coffee at night, want of exercise, unventilated rooms, fiction reading at night.

*TREATMENT*—Feed carefully ; insist upon mental rest. Give warm bath at bed time or hot foot bath with mustard at bed time. Oil should be rubbed to the feet.

*INTERNALLY*—Pippalimul Churna, Jatiphaladi churna or Akarkarbhadi guti at bed time.

In Alopathy Bromide of Potassium, Chloral, Veronal, &c., are given at bed time.

---

## INTESTINAL OBSTRUCTION. *BADDHAN-TRODAR.*

Ch. Chi. Ch. 18,
S. Ni. Ch. 7.

This affection, in which the patient is unable to pass a stool, may commence suddenly as an attack of colic. The constipation not being relieved by medicine; vomiting, first of the contents of the stomach, as partially digested food, then of sour bilious material, and lastly of fœcal matter, occurs; bowels become tender, painful and distended. This affection is caused by accumulations in the interior, stricture, compression, strangulation, altered relation, spasm and paralysis of the intestines.

In the beginning, castor oil or Samudraka Virechan churna to remove constipation. If the patient is strong and robust, Madanadi Vaman churna and Samudrak Virechan churna at the same time.

The belly should be well fomented. A hot bath should also be taken and a large quantity of warm water should be injected several times daily. Thirst might be relieved by washing the mouth with cold water. The patient should be kept quiet and fluid diet should be allowed in small quantities.

Continuous purgatives are useless and harmful.

Experts should be consulted at once, because some times operation is the only cure.

## IRITIS.

It is an inflammation of the iris or that part of the eye in which the round ring of the pupil is formed, and which gives the various colours of the eye. There is intolerance of light, severe stinging pain of the eye and forehead, dull aching in the eye and feverishness. The eye should be protected by a green shade and a darkened room, and fomentation with hot poppy head water should be applied. Leeches may be applied to the temple of the affected eye. (Doctors use atropine solution for the eye).

Arkadi tikdi or Jatiphaladi churna may be given at night. If bowels are costive, Samudrak Virechan churna may be given in the morning.

Treat cause, *e.g.*, Traumatism, syphilis, rheumatism, gout.

## JAUNDICE. *KAMLA.* S. U. Ch. 44. Ch. Chi. Ch. 20

Ascertain and treat cause.

Give warm baths.

*INTERNALLY*—Eliyakadi guti at night and Samudrak Virechan churna in the morning every other day.

Give daily Katurohini churna and Swarjikakshara, or Arogyavardhani and Swarjikakshara, with Nimbadi quath; or Sudarshan churna.

*LOCALLY*—When pain on the side suggests hepatic inflammation, a blister or 4 to 5 leeches applied to the region of the liver will give some relief.

---

## LACTATION. *STANYA.*

S. Sha. Ch. 10.
Ch. Sha. Ch. 8.

*TO INCREASE—INTERNALLY*—Rich foods, *e.g.*, milk, chyavanprash Avaleha; and dill water may be given.

*LOCALLY*—Massage with castor oil.

*TO PURIFY*—Pathadi quath, Haridradi quath or Vachadi quath should be given.

---

## LACTATION FEVER. *STANYOTTHA JWAR.*

*INTERNALLY*—Samshamani guti with Parpat quath after one dose of castor oil.

*LOCALLY*—Hot fomentations to the breast. Massage with Vishagarbha taila. Breasts should be relieved of milk. A wide mouth glass bottle should be filled with hot water, which should be emptied at once; and the bottle to be immediately applied to the breast. Vacuum thus produced will force the milk into the bottle; or breast relievers should be used.

---

## LEPROSY. *MAHAKUSHTHA.*

S. Ni. Ch. 5.
Ch. Chi. Ch. 7.

Perfect cleanliness.

Daily hot baths.

Frequent changes of clothing.

Plentiful and varied diet.

*TREATMENT*—Lohabhasma, Nimbadi quath, Galita-kushtharirasa, Manjishthadi quath, Amrita-bhallatak avaleha, Narsinha churna and Devkusumadi rasa, are all useful, and may be given as desirable.

*VIDANG-TANDUL* Prayoga often cures leprosy.

Bhallatak taila is useful for local application. Chaulmogra oil used internally thrice after meals, may effect cure.

---

## LEUCORRHŒA. *PRADAR (SHWET)* Ch.Chi. Ch. 30.

Improve the general health.

Treat any local cause.

Insist on cleanliness, and abstinence from sexual intercourse.

Treat constipation or any disease of urinary system, if present.

*INTERNALLY*—Pushyanug churna with Darvyadi quath, or Chandraprabha guti with Gooduchi-hima morning and evening, and Pradarariloha gutika with Agnitundi rasa after meals.

*LOCALLY*—Injections (per vaginum) of very hot water, and lotions of Tankanamla, Panchvalkal quath or Jantughna and Grahi tablet (1 in 20 oz. of water). Cotton with glycerine and mayan (galls) kept in the vagina will stop leucorrhœa.

---

## LICHEN-PLANUS. *RAJIKA.* Ash. U. Ch. 31.

Temperate diet, light clothing and cleanliness are necessary.

Baths with Snanraj churna, and then dusting with the churna, are beneficial.

*INTERNALLY*—As an aperient, Samudrak Virechan churna.

*LOCALLY*—If severe, dab the affected parts with the solution of Tutth tikdi (1 tablet in 40 oz. of water).

## LIVER (Congestion of the)—

*SYMPTOMS*—"Coated tongue, bad taste in the mouth, depression of spirits, defective appetite, headache, bowels acting irregularly, stools dark, occasionally bilious diarrhœa, but often constipation, nausea, a sense of weight and fullness in the right side, and pain or uneasiness in the tip of the right shoulder."—*Moore.*

Abstinence in diet and moderate exercise are beneficial.

*INTERNALLY*—Eliyakadi guti at night and Samudrak Virechan churna in the morning. Samshamani guti with Sharpunkha quath before meals, and Arogyavardhani rasa two or three hours after meals.

*LOCALLY*—Mustard leaves should be applied over the liver.

---

## LUMBAGO. *KATIGRAHA-TRIKAGRAHA.* Ch. Su. Ch. 20.

*INTERNALLY*—Castor oil or Shivakshar-pachan in the beginning; if drastic purgative is required, use Ichhabhedi rasa. Agnitundi rasa after meals. If there is fever, Chandraprabha guti, with Gokshura quath, should be given.

*LOCALLY*—Fomentations, Flannel binder, blister, mustard, camphor, capsicum, Turpentine, hot iron, hot oil, Irimedadi taila, Parvativilas taila, and Vishagarbha taila, are all useful and may be used as desired. Massage gives very much relief.

---

## MANIA (Acute). *UNMAD.* S. U. Ch. 62. Ch. Chi. Ch. 14.

Cold water over the head; warm bath and blood letting are useful.

*INTERNALLY*—Jatiphaladi churna or Kanaksundar rasa, to calm excitement.

*CHRONIC*—Narach rasa as purgative, when bowels are costive. Hinguadi ghrit or Lashunadi ghrit, with Saraswat churna, or Medhya Rasayan churna or Brahmi ghrit or Kalyanak ghrit with Hinguadi churna.

*DIET*—Nutritious.

In Alopathy, Chloral Hydrate is preferred in acute mania.

---

**MASTITIS** *STANSHOATH.*

Care in diet.

Samudrak Virechan churna in the morning and Samshamani guti with Parpat quath thrice daily.

*LOCALLY*—Parvativilas taila or Dhatura leaves to be applied as anodyne.

If matter appears to have formed, poultices or hot fomentations should be applied. If the breasts be full, they must be emptied. (See Lactation).

For ulcer, see Ulcer and Fistula.

---

**MEASLES.** *ROMANTIKA.* Madhav.

Careful nursing and rest are necessary.

Give rest in bed at once.

If the bowels are confined, give Samudrak Virechan churna. If there is feverishness, Samshamani guti, and Chandraprabha guti with Parpat quath are best. But if fever rises to 104°, give Tripurbhairav rasa with Parpat quath. If cough continues, Vasaraga or Vasaleha. For thirst, give whey.

*LOCALLY*—Linseed meal poultice or mustard poultice should be applied on the chest, if breathing is hurried.

---

**MELÆNA. (Intestinal Hæmorrhage.)** *RAKTAPITTA-ADHOGAT.* Ch. Chi. Ch. 4. S. U. Ch. 45.

Find source and treat cause, *e.g.*, Dysentery, typhoid, ulcer of the stomach or duodenum, cancer in the intestines, etc.

For the last two causes, in the beginning castor oil should be given, and if it does good, it should be repeated. No food or medicine should be allowed; but only milk with lime water or with Dadimivati if the pain is severe.

Only milk diet is the chief and safest treatment.

---

**MENORRHAGIA.** *ASRAGDAR-RAKTA PRADAR.* S. Sha. Ch. 2. Ch. Chi. Ch.30.

Treat the cause; *e.g.*, Plethora, debility, &c. Insist on rest and perfect quiet. Raise the foot of the bed. Avoid hot drinks and stimulants.

*DIET*—Simple.

If the patient is of a delicate constitution, nutritious food and Chyavanprashavaleh may be given.

Constipation if prevailing previous to the attack, Castor oil or Samudrak Virechan churna should be given before other specific remedies are tried such as, Chandrakala rasa, Ashoka Ghrit, Pushyanug churna, Trifala Churna, Ashokvalkal quath or Karpasmul quath.

In severe cases occurring only at the monthly period, the specific medicines should be begun before eight days; and if the discharge is irregular, they should be continued until the discharge ceases.

*EXTERNALLY*—Cold wet cloths should be laid over the lower part of the bowels and between the thighs

*DURING INTERVALS*—Pradaradiloha guti, Chandraprabha guti or Agnitundi rasa should be given twice after meals. Bowels should be kept open.

An expert of women diseases should be consulted for obstinate menorrhagia.

---

**MUMPS.** *PASHANGARDAB.* S, Ni. Ch. 13.

Rest in bed, warmth, low diet.

*LOCALLY*—Fomentations with hot water or hot poppy head water; Dashang Lep churna during the interval.

*INTERNALLY*—Castor oil or Eliyakadi guti followed, at an interval of three hours, by Samudrak Virechan churna as purgative. Tripurbhairav rasa in small doses with Parpat quath or Samshamani guti for fever and headache.

## NAUSEA. *HRULLAS.* S. U. Ch. 49. Ch. Chi. Ch. 26.

(See vomiting).

Treat the cause, *e.g.*, pregnancy, dyspepsia, worms, &c.

Hot water should be given to drink. Samudrak Virechan churna every day or every other day; and Krimikuthar rasa, with Kapithashtak churna or Hinguadi churna, given every three hours, acts best.

Fruits in diet.

## NEPHRITIS. *URIKKA-SHOATH* Bhai.

See Diet Tables and General Directions.

This is known by the pain in the loins, usually on one side; but on both, if both kidneys are affected. The pain strikes downwards towards the groin, and in males, the testicle is often drawn by spasmodic action of the muscles. The pain is of a dull diffused deep-seated character. The patient lies on his back or perhaps on the affected side, with leg or legs drawn up. The urine is scanty and voided painfully at short intervals; it frequently contains albumen, and often becomes dark from the presence of blood. There is usually considerable feverishness and the bowels are mostly confined.

Perfect rest. A flannel belt next to the skin. Samudrak Virechan churna as a purgative and diaphoretic daily once or twice.

For fever: Tripurbhairav rasa with Parpat quath. For pain, Arkadi, if necessary, at night.

*LOCALLY*—Hot hip bath; mustard poultice on the loins. If convulsions are severe, leeches may be applied.

Barley water; rice water or linseed water may be given to drink.

**NEURALGIA.** *SHOOLA.* S. U. Ch. 42.

Treat if present, syphilis, gout, rheumatism, anæmia or ague. Secure good hygienic conditions. Usually due to retained waste and debility, clean out, therefore, the whole system with Eliyakadi guti at night and Samudrak Virechan in the morning.

Remove debility with Trikatuadi guti and Agnitundi rasa or tonic pills after meals.

For an attack: Internally—Navsagartikdi, Jatiphaladi churna, Lakshminarayan rasa, Akarkarbhadi guti or headache cure may be given.

*LOCALLY*—Hot or cold applications, *e.g.*, solution of Shitaltikdi, Chandanadi taila, Camphor, Irimedadi taila, Vishagarbha taila, or Parvativilas taila may be applied over the part to lessen pain.

---

**NIGHT-BLINDNESS.** *SHLESHMA VIDAGDHA DRISHTI NAKTANDHYA.* S. U. ch. 7.

Castor oil should be dropped into the eyes. Lotion of Shankhadi vati may be dropped into the eyes.

*INTERNALLY*—Saptamrit, Triphala ghrit or Tilvaka ghrita may be given with benefit.

If bowels are constipative, Abhayadi gutika may be given.

---

**OBESITY.** *MEDO-VRIDDHI.* Ch. Su. Ch. 2, Madhav.

(See Diet Tables and General Directions).

Regulation of diet is imperative. Command slow deliberate eating with abundant chewing and no drink with meals or for one to two hours thereafter when water should be freely given. The person should always take exercise, should bathe with Snanraja churna, after a strong massage of oil. Samudrak Virechan churna may be always given in the morning; then Amrita Gugulla guti or Dashang Gugulla guti with Trivritadi quath or Virtarvadi quath should be given three times a day.

*Vidang-tandula prayoga*, also removes obesity.

---

## ORCHITIS. *VRIDDHI.* S. Ni. Ch. 12.

Treat exciting cause, *e. g.*, syphilis, mumps gonorrhœa, etc.

*DURING ATTACK*—Castor oil with milk or Samudrak-virechan churna in the beginning. If vomiting appears necessary, to effect cure Arka churna or Madanadi Vamari churna may be given. Then, it there is fever, Tripurbhairav rasa with Parpat quath three times a day will remove it. Dadimivati guti or Jatiphaladi Churna may be prescribed as anodyne.

*LOCALLY*—Rest, suspensory bandage, pressure by strapping. Vishagarbha taila or Dhatura leaves are useful for application. Paradadi malam or Raskarpuradi taila may be applied to effect resolution.

(Ice and Cologne water are used by doctors).

*During Convalescence*—Vriddhibadhika guti with Vatarirasa or Agnitundi rasa may be given to prevent future attacks.

---

## OTORRHŒA. *KARNA SRAV.* S. U. Ch. 20.

Treat the cause.

Syringe gently with lotion of Jantughna tikdi (1 in 20 oz. of water) or with decoction of Surasadi-gana quath.

*DRY*—Dust in gently powder of Samudrafen or of Tankanamla, then pack the meatus with cotton.

Repeat once or twice daily until the discharge ceases.

**In *chronic cases*,** give internally Kishora Gugul gutika with Sudarshan churna.

**OZÆNA.** *PEENAS.* Ch. Chi. Ch. 26.

Ozæna is the fœtid odour which proceeds from the nose of some people. The fœtor varies in different subjects, but is especially marked when crusts and mucus are expelled and is so intense that a whole ward may be tainted.

*LOCALLY*—Hinguadi taila, Kashisadi taila or bitter almond oil should be dropped in the nose. Daily, nasal douche of Jantughna lotion (1 in 40 of water) or Surastraja lotion (1 in 4 oz. of water). Asperation of very hot saline solution morning and evening, gives excellent results. Peenus Tamaku churna should be given to be used daily as snuff.

*INTERNALLY*—Makshik Bhasma and Praval Bhasma with Sitopaladi churna after meals.

---

**PARALYSIS (Agitans.)** *VEPATHOO.* Ch. Su. Ch. 20. S. Ni. Ch. 1. Madhav.

Rest. Generous diet. Freedom from worry or excitement. (Massage in some cases).

Arogyavardhani rasa or Samshamani guti with Chyavanprasha Avaleha or Abhaya-malaki avaleha in the morning and Saptamrit churna and Agnitundi rasa after meals for debility.

*FOR TREMBLING*—Jatiphaladi churna or Parasik-yavani churna may be given in small doses.

---

**PARALYSIS (Facial).** *ARDIT.* Ch. Chi. Ch. 28. S. Ni. Ch. 1.

May be part of a general paralysis for which see Hemiplegia.

If caused by cold, fomentations with hot poppy head water will cure it.

*INTERNALLY*—Trivritadi churna or Samudrak-virechan churna as a purgative. Improve general health, by tonics, *e.g.*, Mahayograj Gugul gutika, and Agnitundi rasa, and good hygienic conditions.

**PARALYSIS** *ATATVABHI-* Ch. Su. Ch. 19.
**General.)** *NIVESH*

**Weakening of the memory, with delirium, is one of the most characteristic symptoms of general paralysis.**

**According to circumstances, the patient becomes melancholy or else violent; so much so as to strike without reason, the people, who are about him. Sometimes the commencement of the disease reveals itself by apoplectiform or epileptiform attacks, loss of consciousness or transitory hemiplegia. In the second stage, most common form is characterized by delirium of grandeur. The patient lives in a condition of continual satisfaction. He believes himself to be an Emperor, or God. He is possessed of millions, and wishes to distribute them to those, who are around him. His ideas, however, are not like those of monomaniac, ambitious, connected: they are, on the contrary, mobile and contradictory; and whilst the patient is talking to you of his splendour, ask him his calling, and he will artlessly tell you "I am a cobbler."**

**In certain patients hypochondriasis dominates the scene. He believes himself to be dead or fancies that he is persecuted: he refuses all food for fear of poison; he has hallucinations and ideas of suicide.**

**In women, the development of general paralysis most frequently results in irregularity or suppression of menstruation. In its rapid form, the disease may last less than a year. The general duration varies from one to six years.**

**Syphilis is the cause of paralysis general and it is between six and twelve years after the primary infection, that the paralysis general exhibits itself.**

**During the first stage—the patient must avoid fatigue, work and excitement of every kind; a quiet country life, walks in the open air, absolute abstention from alcohol. Give milk diet; laxatives and blisters to the nape of the neck; these are the usual methods.**

If syphilis is found to be responsible, Devkusumadi rasa may be given for a long time. The periods of excitement must be controlled by the use of douche and Arkadi tikdi, Parasikayavani churna, or Akarkarbhadi guti.

(Valerian and Bromides are used in Alopathy).

In a more advanced period, it is generally necessary to place the patient in an asylum, either because the patient becomes dangerous to others or because the melancholia is accompanied by refusal of food and impulse to suicide.

---

## PARAPLEGIA. *URUSTAMBHA*. Ch. Chi. Ch.27

*INTERNALLY*—Yograjgugul guti or Pakshavadhagugul guti, with decoction of Rasnadi quath ; or Pippalyadi churna ; Shad-dharan Yoga churna with Swarjikakshar to clean bowels every other day.

*LOCALLY*—Parvativilasa taila or Vishagarbha taila for massage on the affected part.

---

## PERSPIRATION (Night Sweats.) *PRASVEDA - ATISWEDA.* S. Su, Ch. 24.

Seek cause and treat it.

Change night clothes, if wet.

Hot milk at bed time.

*EXTERNALLY*—Tepid sponging.

*INTERNALLY*—Samudrak-virechan churna in the morning. and Sudarshan churna with Swarjkakshar thrice daily.

For copious Sweats—same treatment.

If fœtid, wash with Snanraj churna.

*INTERNALLY*—Same treatment with more Swarjikakshara.

---

## PERITONITIS. *CHHINNA-ANTRODAR*. Ch. Chi. Ch.18. S. Ni. Ch. 7.

Inflammation of the peritoneum is marked by fever and severe continuous burning pain in the belly increased by pressure. The patient lies on his back in bed with the knees drawn up. If the breathing is watched, it will be seen that the belly is nearly motionless. There is generally costiveness, nausea or vomiting, great prostration of strength, and an anxious expression of countenance. The pulse is frequent and wiry to the touch and the urine is highly coloured. In fatal cases pain increases, the bowels become swollen and tympanitic.

*TREATMENT*—Continued fomentations with hot water over the whole of the body. Enema of warm water should be injected every day. But purgatives should not be administered. Arkadi tikdi in small doses may be given to relieve pain

*DIET*—Fluid.

An early operation is necessary

---

## PHTHISIS. *SHOASH-RAJYAKSHMA.*

S. U. Ch. 41.
Ch. Chi. Ch. 8.

(See Diet Tables and General Directions).

*TREATMENT*—Trikatuadi guti, Navayas tikdi, Suvarna Vasant Malati, Dashang-Abhrak guti or Mrigankvatika guti with Agnitundi rasa or Suvarna Bhasma and Praval Bhasma with Agnitundi rasa after meals for debility. Agnirasa with Vasaleha or Vasaraga for cough and hæmoptysis.

Samshamani guti with decoction of Vidarigandhadigana for fever. Pathadi guti or Dadimivati, with whey for Diarrhœa.

Sitopaladi churna, Talisadi churna or Ashtang Lavan tikdi for anorexia before meals. Chyavanprash Avaleha, Abhayamalaki Avaleha or Agastyaharitaki Avaleha, daily as nutritious food.

*LOCALLY*—mustard or linseed poultice on the chest, if necessary.

---

## PHOSPHATURIA. *KSHAR-MEHA.*

S. Ni. Ch. 6.
Ch. Chi. Ch. 6.

See examination of urine.

Attend to general health; care in diet; mental rest and exercise in open air are beneficial.

Jatiphaladi churna or Arkadi tikdi for insomnia, and Agnitundi rasa with Shankhdrava after meals.

If sugar is found in urine, follow the treatment of diabetes.

If urine is passed in extraordinary quantities, Akarkarbhadi guti or Dadimivati guti may be advantageously given.

---

## PILES-BLEEDING. *RAKTARSHA.*

S. Ni. Ch. 2.
Ch. Chi. Ch. 9.

Treat the cause, *e.g.*, constipation, stricture, &c.

*LOCALLY*—To stop the bleeding, cold water solution of Shital tikdi (or ice where available).

*INTERNALLY*—Nagkeshar with sugar and butter in the morning and Swadishta Virechan churna at night. Jambir raga or Soda water tikdi may be given with Yavakshar to drink.

For dyspeptic patients, Samshamani guti with Kiratadi quath.

Prohibit stimulants and animal food.

Insist on rest and cleanliness.

---

## PILES. *SHUSHKARSHA.*

S. Ni. Ch. 2.
Ch. Chi. Ch. 9.

For pain and inflammation, fomentations or poultices and Ahiphenadi malam to be applied. When there is no pain or inflammation, Kasisadi malam should be applied; or simply cold water.

*INTERNALLY*—Castor oil or Swadishta Virechan churna every day or every other day. If there is feverishness, Samudrak-virechan churna is useful.

If piles protrude after stools, they should be sponged with cold water; cold Surastraja tikdi solution. When they do not return, they must be gently pressed by hand.

Sometimes an operation is necessary.

*DIET*—Simple; milk; whey and Surana (in vegetable).

## Chronic.

Sooranvatak or Ayushyavardhani tikdi after meals; and Swadishta Virechan churna at night. Eliyakadi at night and Samudraka Virechan churna in the morning every four or five days.

Avoidance of capsicum and other such stimulant foods is necessary. Curdled milk, milk and rice and sooran in vegetables, &c., may be taken.

---

## PITYRIASIS. *SIDHMA*. Ch. Chi. Ch. 7. S. Ni. Ch. 5.

*INTERNALLY*—Tricatuadi guti or Mandurloha guti with Nimbadi quath.

*LOCALLY*—Bath with Snanraj churna, and a subsequent application of Snigdha malam.

In chronic cases, Avalgujadi taila is useful, when applied.

*DIET*—Nutritious.

---

## PLAGUE (Bubonic).

Absolute rest in bed; free ventilation; moderate temperature; warmth and stimulation.

For treatment of headache and other symptoms of fever (see Fever).

*EXTERNALLY*—Mustard plasters or blisters over the bubo.

*DIET*—Fluid: Chiefly milk frequently and in small quantities.

*INTERNALLY*—Samudraka-virechan churna in the beginning. Diaphoretics are beneficial. The patient's strength should be sustained by Agnitundi rasa.

---

## PLEURISY.

This is inflammation of the *serious* membrane covering the outside of the lungs, and lining the *inside* of the chest.

At the commencement of acute pleurisy, there is, generally, shivering followed by 'fever' and by pain or stitch, in some part of the chest. This in a few hours becomes acute stabbing pain and is generally most felt in the side about the level of the nipple, shooting to the front of the chest to the collar bone, or to the armpit. There is short dry cough, the breathing is short and catching. The pulse is frequent and hard. If not checked, dropsy of the chest results.

*TREATMENT*—The patient should be kept in bed, warm and free from draughts. He should move and talk as little as possible. Hot linseed or mustard poultices may be applied over the chest. Hot poppyhead poultices should be applied over the painful part. Leeches are also desirable and may be applied.

*INTERNALLY*—Arkadi tikdi every two hours in 3 or 4 gr. doses.

During convalescence, protection against cold and chill is urgently necessary; and if there is any remaining cough, it may be treated with Vasavaleha.

## PNEUMONIA. *RAKTASTHIVI-SANNIPAT.* Bhav.

*SYMPTOMS*—Usually it commences as a severe cold with chills and high fever. There is a short dry cough, with scanty tenacious expectoration at first white and frothy; at a later period rusty or streaked with blood. Respiration is rapid and short, rising from the normal fourteen or sixteen to thirty or more, while body temperature rises to 104° or 105°.

*TREATMENT*—Insist on entire rest.

*INTERNALLY*—Samudrak-virechan churna in the beginning. Chandraprabha guti with Vacha churna or Arka churna to reduce temperature; Angitundi rasa every four hours for debility.

For cough and other symptoms of chest, Agni-rasa and Navasagar with Vasaraga.

*LOCALLY*—Poultices on the chest. At night a jacket of cotton wool should be lightly tied over the chest and back. The atmosphere of the chamber should be maintained moist and at an equable temperature. To effect this, the steam from a kettle of water boiled in a distant corner of the room, may be allowed to escape into the room.

## PREGNANCY. *SAGARBH-AVASTHA.*

S. Sha. Ch. 10.
Ch. Sha. Ch. 8.

Generally, drugs are not administered to pregnant women; but for dangerous diseases it is better to consult a good well-experienced physician and treat accordingly, with care.

If nausea and vomiting are severe, Samshamani-g uti may be given every day.

If bowels are constipative, castor oil may be given twice a week.

## PROLAPSUS ANI. *GUDA-BHRANSHA.*

S. N. Ch. 13.
Ch. Chi. Ch. 10.

Treat the cause, *e.g.*, debility, worms, phimosis, stricture, &c.

*INTERNALLY*—Changaeri ghrit, Chavyadi ghrit, or Swadisht Virechan churna.

*LOCALLY*—Solution of Jantughna and Grahi tikdi (1 in 10 oz. of water) should be applied. Solution of Kasis tikdi (1 in 2 oz. of water) should be injected.

Support should be given to the anus.

## PROSTATE GLAND (Enlargement of) *ASTHILA* (*Mutraghat*)

S. U. Ch. 58.

The prostrate gland surrounds the urethra at the neck of the bladder; the most important disease of this gland is slow enlargement most common in old men characterized by frequent calls to make water, especially during the night, increasing slowness and difficulty in making water and straining.

Irregular diet, fatigue and exposure to cold should be avoided; the bowels should be kept open. Enema of warm water will prove beneficial.

If the urine is acid, give Hinguadi guti; and if the urine is acid, ropy and thick, give Hinguadi guti with Mutra-virechan quath and Parasik Yavani churna. But if it is alkaline, thick and ropy, Trayodashang Guggul guti and Mutra-virechan quath with Yavakshar. If the liver be not acting well, Yavakshar, especially, should be given. Peculiarly shaped catheter is sometimes necessary. Consult some expert in serious cases.

(See Examination of Urine).

## PRURITUS and PRURIGO. *ALASAK-RAKASA.* S. Ni. Ch. 5. Ch. Chi. Ch. 7.

Treat the cause. Always examine urine for sugar. Avoid stimulants. The skin should be kept clean.

*EXTERNALLY*—Cold lotion of Shital tikdi or ice-cold water is best for local application. Bath with Snanraj with vigorous rubbing. When troublesome itching occurs, Snigdha malam should be applied.

*INTERNALLY*—Samudrak Virechan churna in the beginning as a purgative, then Kishor Gugul guti, or Lohagugul guti with Manjishthadi quath should be given three times a day.

## PRURITUS ANI. *AHIPUTNA.* S. Ni. Ch. 13.

Always carefully examine anus and rectum. Treat rectal ulcer, fissure, worms; prohibit tobacco, coffee and alcohol. Diet—very careful, if gouty. Insist on extreme cleanliness.

*INTERNALLY*—Swadishta Virechan churna or Samudrak-virechan churna, with Patoladi quath.

*LOCALLY*—Thorough washing with solution of Jantughna and Grahitikdi (1 in 10 oz. of water) or Kanduprashaman quath; then Rasanjan or Kashisadi taila should be applied.

(See Fissure of the Anus and Ulcer).

## PRURITUS VULVAE. *YONIKANDU.* Ch. Chi. Chi. 30 S. U. Ch. 38.

Examine urine for sugar. Treat diabetes, gout, etc.

*TREATMENT*—Internally—Chandraprabhaguti with Patoladi quath, and Swarjikakshar.

*LOCALLY*—Sponging with hot water or hot solution of Surastraja tablet, Tankanamla tikdi, Jantughna and Grahi tablet (1 in 10 oz. of water); Panchvalkal quath or Jantughna tablet (1 in 24 oz. of water,); then dusting with Tankanamla powder (Boric acid); or Kandu Prashaman churna.

---

## PSORIASIS. *VICHARCHIKA.* S. Ni. Ch. 5. Ch. Chi. Ch. 7.

Begins as small round shining itching spots, soon becoming covered with thin white scales; which falling off, leave the skin beneath slightly tender and reddened. The spots increase in size but retain the circular shape, until they attain several inches in circumference, when they become broken, and assume the form of irregular scaly patches. It attacks frequently the inner surface of the thigh and armpits, the palms of the hands and the nails.

*TREATMENT*—Avoid all articles of diet which induce dyspepsia. If constipation present, remove it with Samudrak-virechan churna. Narayanjwarankush rasa with Arkadi quath, Chopchini quath, or Chopchiniadi churna, should be given twice a day after meals. If syphilitic, Devkusumadi rasa will cure it.

*EXTERNALLY*—Vachadi lepa, Gandhak malam or Paradadi malam is useful for application.

In chronic cases, baths with Gandhak water (Gandhak in water) will aid relief.

---

## RETENTION of URINE. *VAT-BASTI.* S. U. Ch. 58.

Treat the cause, *e.g.*, paraplegia, enlarged prostrate, gonorrhœa, stricture, worms, hæmorrhoids

Retention may be present with and indicated by incontinence and constant dribbing.

*LOCALLY*—Hot baths, fomentations or leeches to perinæum, if necessary.

*INTERNALLY*—Akarkarbhadi guti, Arkadi tikdi, Jatiphaladi churna or Kanaksundar rasa may be given as an anodyne, when required.

Catheter is often required to draw out the urine.

---

## RHEUMATISM. *SANDHIGAT-VATROGA AMVAT.*

Ch. Chi. Ch. 28. Madhav.

See Diet Tables and General Directions.

The pain generally comes on in one of the larger joints, which is highly inflamed, red and swollen, so that it cannot be moved, and the slightest touch is shrunk from. It commences usually after exposure to damp or cold with fever, a full quick pulse; hot skin, coated tongue, and scanty urine, which deposits a dusky reddish sediment. The inflammation may attack several or all the joints, but more commonly two or three are affected one day, and then others are suddenly attacked; the first joint implacated growing, almost as suddenly, comparatively well. There are also frequent characteristic sour perspirations. The duration of the disease may be a fortnight to three weeks. Acute rheumatism is more common in young than in old persons, and from its tendency to affect the heart, must always be regarded as serious.

*Chronic Rheumatism* is most frequent in elderly persons. There is pain in larger joints accompanied sometimes with swelling: there is generally neither fever nor perspiration.

*TREATMENT*—Keep patient at rest and clothe him in flannel. Clothes well saturated with hot poppyhead water, or with hot water, in which Swarjikskar has been dissolved, should be well wrapped round the parts; and then be covered with oiled silk or waterproof cloth. Vishagarbha taila may also be applied.

*INTERNALLY*—Castor oil or Samudrak-virechan churna should be given to move the bowels; then Yavakshar should be given 4 times a day with Punarnavadi quath, Rasanadi quath or Mutravirechan quath, or Pippalyadi churna may be given 4 times a day with Gokshuradi guti. Tripurbhairav rasa with Parpat quath may be given to lessen fever and pain. If there is sleeplessness from pain, Arkadi tikdi may be given at night.

In Alopathy, Salicylate of soda is considered specific for rheumatism.

*DIET*—Milk and rice.

Whenever water may be given to drink, it must first be mixed with Swarjikakshar.

### Chronic Rheumatism.

Warm clothing, generous living, rubbing the parts with Vishagarbha taila, and Arkadi tikdi internally, occasionally at night constitute all the treatment.

---

## RINGWORM of the body. *DADROO,* S. Ni. Ch. 5. Ch. Chi. Ch. 7.

Wash with carbolic soap and water twice a day and then rub Dadrughna Malam thoroughly into the affected part. In chronic cases, the skin must be well washed with hot water, soap and scrubbing brush, and then Dadrughna malam should be rubbed in; or Avalgujadi lepa, Lakshadi lepa or Kushtadi lepa with whey may be tried.

Insist on cleanliness.

*INTERNALLY*—Samshamani gutika with Nimbadi quath may be given.

---

## RINGWORM of the scalp. *INDRALUPTA.* S. Ni. Ch. 13 Ch. Su. Ch. 3.

*LOCALLY*—If extensive, shave the head: if in a few places only, clearly mark out every patch, wash with carbolic soap, and extract the diseased hair. Then the affected part should be rubbed over vigorously with Paradadi malam or Dadrughna malam. When the fungus has disappeared, apply Chandanadi taila over the head.

Diet should be liberal. Constipated bowels should be relieved and tonics such as Tonic Pills, Saptamrit churna or Samshamani guti should be given.

---

## SCABIES. *PAMA-KATCHHOO.*

S. Ni. Ch. 5.
Ch. Chi Ch. 7.

Examine for Albuminaria during treatment.

The parts affected should be first well washed with carbolic soap and water, and then well rubbed with Paradadi malam, Gandhak malam, Turushkadi malam or Adityapak taila, twice daily.

*INTERNALLY*—Gandhak rasayan with Shiva churna or Swadishta-virechan churna and Samshamani guti. Give Chandraprabha guti if there is albuminaria.

---

## SCIATICA. *GRIDHRASI.*

S. Ni. Ch. 1.
Ch. Chi. Ch. 28.

Sciatica is a painful affection of the large nerve, passing down the back of the thigh. There is acute agonising pain extending from the buttock to the ham.

*REST*—Warm flannel round the part. Hot fomentations, ironing the part with hot flat iron after spreading flannel or a layer of cotton wool over it. Mustard poultices or small blisters over the more painful parts.

*INTERNALLY*—Bowels should be kept open with Swadista-virechan churna or Samudrak-virechan churna. In a case, connected with rheumatism the treatment of chronic rheumatism should be followed. Rasanadi-gugul gutika or Swayambhoo-gugul guti with Rasanadi quath will prove effective.

For pain, Vatarirasa and Jatiphaladi churna are useful internally; and Vishgarbha taila or Parvativilas taila for external application.

*DIET*—Nutritious, *e.g.*, Chyavanprash avaleh or Abhayamalaki avaleh.

## SCROFULA. *GANDAMALA-APACHI.* S. Ni. Ch. 11. Ch. Chi. Ch. 17.

Good air, good food, Agastya-haritaki avaleha and exercise may prevent its active manifestation.

*INTERNALLY*—Castor oil, when necessary. Kishor-gugul guti or Kanchnar-gugul guti with Manjishthadi quath three times a day, to be continued for a long time. If the patient is syphilitic, Devkusumadi rasa with Chopchini quath. If anæmic, Trikatuadi guti or Punarnava-mandur guti after meals.

*LOCALLY*—Doshaghna lepa, Chakramarda taila or Gunjadi taila.

For ulcers, Jatyadi Ghrita or malam locally, and Triphala-gugul guti internally.

---

## SINUS. *NADI-VRINA.* S. Ni. Ch. 10.

Requires operation.

Fomentations with hot water or poultices to the inflamed part at first. After operation, Tiladi lepa should be applied on the part like a poultice.

Wash the wound with Panchvalkal quath or solution of Jantughna and Grahi tikdi (1 in 10 oz. of water). Fill it with Jatyadi malam.

*INTERNALLY*—Kanchnar-gugul guti, Devkusumadi rasa, or Trifala-gugul guti with Manjishthadi quath.

---

## SMALL-POX. *MASOORIKA.* S. Ni. Ch. 13. Ch. Chi. Ch. 17.

The patient should, as much as possible, be isolated, if practicable in a separate building.

The bowels should be kept moderately open by Ashwakanchuki guti or Samudrak-virechan churna. The legs and arms may be sponged daily with warm water.

*DIET*—Fluid, consisting mostly of milk.

The patient should be prevented from scratching, and if a child, the hands should be muffled. Itching and irritation may be relieved by applying warm ghee, cold butter or Snigdh malam on the parts, by sprinkling the parts with Jasatpushpa (zinc oxide).

During the drying up period, Samshamani guti, three times a day, and Vasaraga in case of cough internally.

Observe perfect cleanliness by frequent changes of clothing, and if the patient is not very weak, a daily bath. If the patient is very weak, two beds should be kept to change clothes.

---

## SPASTIC PARAPLEGIA. *KALAYAKHANJ.* S. Ni. Ch. 1.

*SYMPTOMS*—The patient staggers, particularly when commencing to walk; he cannot walk firmly without support. He lifts his feet unnecessarily high, throws them forwards and outwards, and brings the heels down with a stamp. When walking in the dark, he probably falls.

*INTERNALLY*—Trikatuadi guti and Agnitundi rasa or Tonic pills after meals. Pakshwadha-gugul guti with Rasanadi quath morning and evening.

If due to syphilis, give Devkusumadi rasa.

*LOCALLY*—Massage with Vishagarbha taila.

*DIET*—Nutritious and easily digestible. Abhayamalaki or Chyavanprash with milk.

---

## SPERMATORRHŒA. *SHUKRAMEHA.* S. Ni. Ch. 6. Ch. Chi. Ch. 6.

Ascertain the cause and remove it. If the prepuce is long it should be removed. If masturbation is the cause, stop it. If bowels are confined, they should be opened by Shiva churna, Trivritadi churna or Samudrak-virechan churna. Agnitundi rasa or Ashwagandhadi churna with Shukrashodhana-gana churna, are useful. Chandraprabha guti with Praval Bhasma also proves curative.

Ascertain Spermatorrhœa by examination of urine. (See sexual debility and nocturnal emissions).

## SPLENIC ENLARGEMENT. *PLIHODAR.* Ch. Chi. Ch. 18. S. Ni. Ch. 7.

Treat ague if present.

*INTERNALLY*—Samudraka Virechan churna, every other day with other medicines, if bowels are costive. Arogyavardhani rasa and Samshamani guti or Sudarshan churna with Sharpunkha quath every morning and evening; Mandura Loha guti with Agnitundi rasa or Tonic pills after meals.

In cases of spleen becoming suddenly painful, hot fomentations should be applied on the part.

*DIET*—Milk or curdled milk and rice.

## SPRUE. *GRAHNI.* S. U. Ch. 40. Ch. Ch. Ch. 19.

*SYMPTOMS*—The symptoms are peculiar and consist at first of, often painless diarrhœa, occurring chiefly in the early morning. The stools passed are light, sometimes of white colour, often exactly like chalk and water and generally copious, and frothy. As the disease advances, light stools are also passed in the evening or soon after meals. The calls to stool are urgent. The most distressing symptoms are distention of the bowels by flatus, eructations having a rotten odour, and other dyspeptic symptoms. The pulse is feeble, and the tongue furred in the centre. The patient generally confesses to a feeling of uneasiness about the liver. If this condition be not checked the person falls into a state of confined weakness, or cachexia. The stools become more numerous; emaciation takes place. Then probably stools become dysenteric, and the patient dies exhausted.

Care in diet is the chief treatment; the diet should wholly consist of sour fruits, *popaiya*, previously boiled milk, or whey, to be taken every hour or every two hours in small proportions.

In bad cases, only whey should be given frequently, and in as much quantity, as can be conveniently taken during the whole day with Jirak and salt, or Ashtanglavana tikdi.

*TREATMENT*—Yavakshara, Swarjikakshara or Pippaliadi churna should be given in small doses, before food. Every 4 to 6 days, castor oil may be given. If there is no improvement by this treatment, change of climate is advisable. During the above treatment, some specific should be given at least once for round worms (See Worms).

If further treatment is desired, give Dadimashtak churna, Kapitthshtak churna or Hinguashtak churna for anorexia. Ambashthadi quath or Bhoonimbadi churna for dyspepsia; Panchamrit Parpati rasa, Arogyavardhani rasa, Grahanikapat rasa or Arkadi tikdi for diarrhœa and Shankhvati tikdi for colic.

Carefully examine teeth and keep them perfectly clean. Teeth and gums should be washed every time after taking food with astringent and antiseptic solutions.

## STIFF NECK. *MANYA-STAMBH.* S. Ni. Ch. 1.

*TREATMENT*—The neck should be rubbed with Narayan taila or Vishagarbha taila and it should be fomented. Stiff neck is relieved also by spreading flannel or a layer of cotton wool over the part and then ironing with a hot flat iron.

*INTERNALLY*—Yograjgugulu guti or Chandraprabha guti or Pippalyadi churna should be given with Rasanadi quath.

Flannel should be wrapped round the neck.

## STOMATITIS. *MUKHROGA-MUKHPAK.* Ch. Chi. Ch. 26. S. Ni. Ch. 16.

Care in diet is imperative.

Treat dyspepsia, if present.

The teeth should be looked after. Bowels should be kept open by castor oil, Shivaksharapachan churna or Samudrakvirechan churna.

*LOCALLY*—Wash the mouth two or three times daily with a solution of Jantughna and Grahi tablet ( 1 in 10 oz. of water), Panchvalkal quath or solution of Surashtraja tablet. Gargle with Irimedadi taila. Application of Irimedadi taila in the mouth gives relief. Khadiradi guti should be kept in the mouth and allowed to be dissolved slowly. Give Agnitundi rasa after meals.

---

## STYE. *ANJANANAMIKA.* S. U. Ch. 3.

*LOCALLY*—Should be frequently well fomented with hot water, permitted to come to a head, and then pricked with lancet or neddle to let the 'matter' out. Rubbing with Rasanjan or Shiladichurna on the part is sometimes beneficial.

*INTERNALLY*—Rasayan Churna or Saptamrit Churna to remove general debility.

---

## SUNSTROKE. *SURYABHIGHATJANYA MOORCHHA.* S. U Ch. 46.

Frequently previous to an attack of sunstroke, the person affected becomes irritable, restless, and complains of headache. He feels dull and listless. The appetite fails and a feeling of nausea with constipation is often present. An absence of perspiration may also be noticed; the skin may be unusually hot and dry and there may be a slight sensation of giddiness. Either after the foregoing premonitory symptoms or without them, heat fainting commences with feelings of faintness, sickness, giddiness, shivering, cold extremities; frequent desire to make water and sometimes drowsiness. The face is pale, the surface of the body is cold, the breathing is of a sighing character; the action of the heart and pulse is weak; the pupils of the eyes are dilated and there may be more or less insensibility.

*TREATMENT*—Cold water or cold lotion of Shital tikdi (or ice) to chest, back and abdomen. Punkhas should be used to cool the surrounding atmosphere. If the body is too hot, it should be covered with wet clothes. The extremities should be rubbed ; mustard poultice should be applied to the nape of the neck. If fainting is prolonged, leeches may be applied at the roots of the hair above the temples.

## SYNOVITIS of knee-joints. *KROSHTRUK-SHIRSH.* S. Nl. Ch. 1.

Inflammation of synovial membrane of the knee joints. It is attended with pain, especially on movement and with swelling of the joint.

For *Acute* disease—See Rheumatism.

For *Chronic*—Samudrak Virechan churna every other day and Yograj Gugul guti or Lohagugula guti with Trivritadi quath, three times a day, for a few days. Chandraprabha guti may also be given with advantage.

*LOCALLY*—Wrap the part in cotton wool.

Doshaghna lepa, petroleum, Vishagarbha taila or Datura leaves are useful as an application.

Leeches may be applied, if necessary.

## SYPHILIS. *FIRANG.* Bhav.

*INTERNALLY*—Devkusumadi rasa or Updanshahara guti No. 1 with Manjishthadi quath or Sariva quath every morning and evening: Manduraloha guti with Agnitundi rasa or Updanshahara guti No. 2 after meals for debility.

*LOCALLY*—Wash with Panchvalkal quath, Jantughna and Grahi lotion tablet (1 in 10 oz. of water) and then apply Paradadi malam, Turushkadi malam or Jatyadi malam.

*DIET*—Nutritious: bread and milk.

Soft chancre—Destroy the *Chancre* with a strong caustic, *e.g.*, Tuttha tikdi and apply Paradadi malam or Kasisadi malam.

A *syphilitic infant* should be brought up by hand; and should be treated with Saptasalivati guti and Samshamani guti; and Rasakarpuradi taila (2 p.c.) or Paradadi malam with three parts of oil to be applied to sores where they appear.

## TETANUS. *DHANUSTAMBH.* S. Ni. Ch. 1. Ch. Chi. Ch. 28.

*SYMPTOMS*—The disease usually commences with stiffness of the neck and about the jaws, which are opened and closed with difficulty. There is often difficulty of swallowing leading to violent ejection of fluids from the mouth or through the nose. In the course of a few hours or days, the jaws become firmly closed. Spasms of the limbs and body also supervene, by which the patient may be bent like a bow. The face is contorted into a frightful grin. There is agonising pain in the limbs. The muscles remain hard and do not thoroughly relax, unless the patient sleeps.

A cut, scratch or wound somewhere in the body is the seat of the poison..

*TREATMENT*—Keep the patient in a dark room and in perfect quiet. Clean away all blood and foreign bodies which may be in the wound; then wash it with lotion of Jantughna tikdi (1 in 20 oz. of water); and then dust with Tankanamla churna (Boric acid).

*INTERNALLY*—Lakshminarayan rasa, Dadimivati guti, or Jatiphaladi churna may be given.

*LOCALLY*—Heat to spine.

**For Infantile Tetanus**—The jaws must be gently separated by the end of a spoon, protected by a small piece of linen rolled round it, then milk diluted in one-third the quantity of lime water, should be given every hour as much as the child can swallow. A warm bath should be given twice daily and an enema; half milk, half lime water should be given thrice daily. Samshamani one pill and Lakshminarayan rasa one grain every six hours will bring relief.

---

## TEETHING. *DANTOADBHEDA.* Asht.

Sixty grs. of Swarjikakshara well mixed with one ounce of honey, or Pippalyadi Pratisarana with honey should be well rubbed on the gums two or three times daily; gums should be lanced if necessary. Almost any variety of skin disease may occur during dentition, but rarely needs much medical treatment. Only the parts affected should be kept perfectly clean, by washing daily with Snanaraj after which, oil, crem or Snigdh malam should be applied. For constipation and flatulence, castor oil and dill water should be given. For diarrhœa, see Diarrhœa. For cough, Vishadi churna with honey. For debility, Samshamani pills.

---

## THIRST. *TRISHA.* Ch. Su. Ch. 24. S. U. Ch. 48

Is a symptom of disease, and is always an accompaniment of fevers; also attends certain forms of dyspepsia, and is a prominent symptom of diabetes.

Treat cause: give Jambirraga or Samudrak Virechan churna if diabetes: Swarjikakshara or Soda water tablets if dyspeptic: Trishna Prashamana quath if fever (see Fever).

---

## TONSILITIS. *GALAGRIHA-KANTHA-SHALOOKA.* Ch Su. Ch. 17. S. Ni. Ch. 16.

For mild cases, externally: Hot fomentations or mustard poultice, and gargle with Surashtraja tikdi solution. Internally: give Eliyakadi guti at night and Samudrak virechan churna in the morning.

When the tonsils gather, fomentation should be used outside; the throat should be frequently steamed and Devkusumadi rasa should be given internally with the above-named purgative. When there is ulceration, concentrated solution of Surashtraja tablet (1 in ½ oz. of water) should be applied.

**Chronic Tonsilitis**—Avoid cold and chill. Remove all carious teeth, gargle with Triphala quath or Panchvalkal quath. Apply Triphala churna with honey (or glycerine).

*INTERNALLY*—Tonic pills or Mandurloha guti after meals.

*DIET*—Nutritious.

## TOOTH-ACHE. *DANTROAGA.* S. Ni. Ch. 16.

*INTERNALLY*—Samudrak Virechan churna as purgative at first: then Dadimivati guti or headache cure tablet as anodyne.

*LOCALLY*—Rub the gum with Navsagar and the teeth with Dantmanjan. Apply hot fomentations to inside of the mouth. Gargle with Irimedadi taila. Oil of cloves, oil of cinnamon or opium water (½ gr. opium in ½ dr. of water) applied on cotton wool to the teeth gives relief. When there is a large hollow in the tooth, it should be filled up with paste of Vidang churna and bees wax. Clean the teeth after each meal.

---

## TYMPANITIS. *ADHMAN.* S. Ni. Ch. 1. Ch Chi. Ch. 28.

Give initially Shivakshar-pachan churna: Dviruttar-hinguadi churna: Shad-dhraan churna: Shiva churna: or Vaishvanar churna with Swarjikakshar; if with colic, add Shankhvati tikdi. When these medicines do not produce the desired effect, and also if symptoms of cholera and sprue appear, give Krimikuthar rasa, which will be found invaluable.

**For Infants**, Shringyadi churna with castor oil and dill water are best.
*LOCALLY*, Fomentations on the part, enema, &c.
*DIET*—milk, barley, rice, &c. with Dhanyak-Jirak churna.

---

## ULCERS. *VRINA.* S. Su. Ch. 22. Ch. Chi. Ch.13.

Treat the cause, *e.g.*, syphilis, tubercle, gout. Insist upon rest in bed.

*INTERNALLY*—Amritagugul guti, Kishorgugul guti or Triphalagugul guti with Manjisthadi quath or Varunadi quath.

*LOCALLY*—Fomentations with hot water or poultices, for a time in the beginning; then if the ulcer is superficial, wash it with lotion of Jantughna tikdi (1 in 24 oz. of water), Triphala water, or Panchvalkal quath, and then dust it with Jasat pushpa, Boric acid, Tankanamla powder or

Lodhradi churna. If the ulcer is deep, after washing it with the above lotion, dress it with gauze smeared with Jatyadi taila or Chandanadi Taila daily; but if the ulcer is large and not very deep, Jatyadi malam, Kasisadi malam or Paradadi malam should be applied daily. All kinds of ulcers should be bandaged after dressing. Ulcers should never be kept open. (See Vrana Vidhi).

## URIC ACID-DIATHESES. *SIKATA-MEHA.* S. Ni. Ch. 6. Ch. Chi. Ch. 6.

The urine of persons passing red or pink gravel is clear, acid, of dark golden colour, and often less abundant than the urine of health. After it has cooled, the red or pink deposit appears as a sediment. Hearth-burn, acidity of the stomach, and other symptoms of indigestion or disordered liver are present. Headacho and depression are also present.

For treatment see *Calculi Renal.*

## URTICARIA. *SHEETA-PITTA.* Madhav.

Regulate diet. Prevent scratching. If the stomach is full and nausea felt, give Madanadivaman churna as an emetic. If drastic purgative is required, Ichhabhedi rasa, or Narach rasa should be given; otherwise Eliyakadi guti followed after two hours by Samudrak Virechan churna. For repeated attacks Rewanchitwak with Swarjikakshar, or Sudarshan churna with Swarjika-kshar may be given for a few days. Bath with hot water with a solution of Swarjika kshar dissolved 1 oz. in 1 gallon of water will bring relief.

## VOMITING. *CHHARDI.* S. U. Ch. 49. Ch. Chi. Ch. 23.

Ascertain whether there is any source of peripheral irritation, such as intestinal, renal or biliary colic; exclude peritonitis, intestinal obstruction, hernia, renal disease, cerebral tumor, etc.

Regulate the diet and treat dyspepsia. Give internally Sodawater tablet with very cold water or ice to check vomiting. Avipattiker tikdi, Shivakshar-pachan churna or Samudrak Virechan churna for free action of bowels. Eladichurna will often cure vomiting. If accompanied by colic, give Shankhvati.

*LOCALLY*—Counter-irritants on the epigastrium, *e.g.*, mustard poultice.

*DIET*—Shalyodan; cocoanut water: whey: grapes: pomegranate juice, prevents vomiting.

## WARTS. *MASHAK.* S Ni. Ch. 13.

Frequently when left alone, they gradually disappear. When warts grow with a thin neck, a piece of strong waxed thread or horse hair may be tied tightly round the narrow part, when the wart will fall off. Lotion of Surastraja tikdi or Tuttha tikdi, if applied for a few days, will remove most warts.

After falling off of the warts, the part should be touched with Surastraja tikdi lotion for a few days.

## WHOOPING COUGH.

Fresh air, good food. If feverish, give rest in bed. During the paroxysms of cough, the child's back should be rubbed with Vishgarbha taila and opium.

*INTERNALLY*—Krimikuthar rasa or Arkadi tikdi with Vasaraga. If there is feverishness and tendency to bronchitis, the patient should be kept warm: the head should be kept well raised on pillows at night and the windows of the room should be open avoiding draughts. Devadhupa (storax) should be burnt in the room, three or four times a day. Doctors give for inhaling 1 oz. of carbolic acid in 14 oz. of water. For subsequent debility, Samshamani and Mandur-vatak tikdi are useful.

## WORMS. *KRIMI.* S. U. Ch. 54. Ch. Su. Ch. 19.

**For Tape Worms**—Remove mucus from intestine by Samudrak-virechan churna. Give low diet, milk, &c., for two days. Then give Krimimudgar rasa with Triphaladi quath or Vidangchurna, or Vidangsaravaleha guti followed by castor oil.

**Round Worms**—Tiktajirak churna, Kirman: churna, Krimimudgar rasa with Triphaladi quath or Krimighna tikdi.

**Thread Worms**—Regulate the diet and insist upon salt with food. *Internally*, give tonic pills or Vidangadyavaleha, after meals, and Samudrak-virechan churna in the morning.

# QUATHS.

## General Instructions for preparing Quaths.

Take about ½ to 2 tolas of coarse powder of quath and add water 16 times its proportion. Boil and make it into a decoction. When one fourth the quantity of water is evaporated, strain the remaining portion and prescribe the same to the patient. It would be convenient to prepare the quath in several doses for the whole day. But under no circumstances keep the decoction overnight. Always prepare fresh quaths.

Generally the quaths are prescribed as **Anupans** of other drugs. The principal drug should, therefore, be taken or mixed with such decoction.

The **dose** given below is for the **coarse powder** only.

The prices quoted are for ¼ lb. packets of coarse powders of quaths.

### Abhayadi Quath.

Sha. M. Ch. 2 V. 35.

Dose ½ to 2 tolas, to be taken twice a day. Chief ingredients are Abhaya, Musta, Dhanyaka, Raktachandan, Padmaka, Indrayava, Gudoochi, Patha, Katuki, etc. Alterative, bitter tonic and slightly laxative. Specially useful in long continued fevers: restores lost appetite, removes chronic constipation, and cures cough and other like complications of fever. It is also used in pneumonia.

### Ambasthadi-gana Quath.

S. Su. Ch. 38.

Dose ½ to 2 tolas, to be taken twice a day. Chief ingredients are Patha, Lodh a, Bilvapeshika, Dhatakipushpa, Palasha, Padma, Keshara Astringent, demulcent, bitter tonic, diuretic. A very useful remedy for diarrhœa, dysentery, dyspepsia and catarrhal affections of genito-urinary system such as gonorrhœa, cystitis and leucorrhœa.

**Amritadi Quath.** Bang

Dose ½ to 2 tolas, to be taken twice a day. Chief ingredients are Gudoochi, Musta, Kirata and Shunthi. Bitter tonic, stomachic, stimulant. Useful in indigestion, anorexia, and torpid liver with constipation. Use with Soda Bicarb. in hyperacidity.

**Arkadi Quath.** Ni. Part. II.

Dose ½ to 2 tolas, to be taken twice a day. Chief ingredients are Arka, Jiraka, Trikatu, Kantakarika, Shringi, Kushta, etc. Alterative, stimulant and expectorant. Useful in dengue fever, acute bronchitis, pneumonia and fevers complicated with chest affections.

**Arjunatwak Quath.**

Dose 20 to 40 grs. To be taken twice a day. Astringent and tonic. Useful in cirrhosis, scrofula and heart diseases.

**Kalingakadi Quath.**

Ch. Chi. Ch. II

Dose ½ to 2 tolas. To be taken twice a day. Chief ingredients are Indrayava, Patola and Katuki. Bitter tonic, anti-periodic. Useful in fevers generally and specially suitable in malarial fever with liver complaints.

**Kiratadi Quath.**

Ch. Chi. Ch 3

Dose ½ to 2 tolas to be taken twice a day. Bitter tonic, anti-periodic. Cures atonic dyspepsia, is highly useful in malaria and other fevers. Chief ingredients are Kirata, Musta, Gudoochi, Patha, Shunthi, etc.

## Gudoochyadi Quath.

Ch. Chi. Ch. 3

Dose ½ to 2 tolas to be taken twice a day. Chief ingredients are Gudoochi, Saptaparnatwak, Kirata and Shunthi. Bitter tonic. Stomachic and anti-periodic. Used in anorexia, alcoholism, chyluria, dyspepsia, dysentery, malaria, etc. The chief ingredient of this quath, the Saptaparnatwak is an anti-periodic like quinine without its bad after-effect.

## Chopchini Quath.

Dose 1 to 3 tolas, to be taken twice a day like tea, with churna of twak and some sugar. Diaphoretic, stimulant, alterative and resolvent. Useful in rheumatism, gout, epilepsy, general cachexia, scrofula and seminal weakness. This is much used by Vaidyas and Hakims in constitutional tertiary syphilis. Should be continued for a long time.

## Trishnaprashamana Quath.

Ch. Su. Ch. 4.

Dose ½ to 2 tolas, to be taken three times a day. Chief ingredients are Shunthi, Dhanvayasa, Parpat, Kirata, Gudoochi, Patola, Dhanya, Chandana, etc. Bitter tonic, stomachic. Specially suitable for thirst due to dyspepsia or fever; allays thirst; cures dyspepsia and strengthens appetite.

## Triphala Quath.

Sha. M. Ch. 2. V. 118.

Dose ½ to 2 tolas. Contains Abhaya, Amalaka and Bibhitaka. Astringent. Externally it is used as a wash in ulcers. Filtered water of this quath is also used as eye wash in eye diseases.

## Triphaladi Quath.

Sha. M. Ch. 2

Dose ½ to 2 tolas, to be taken twice a day

10 tola packet.

with Vidang churna. Chief ingredients are Triphala, Deodar, Musta, Shigrutwak, etc. Alterative, laxative. Recommended for worms.

**Trivritadi Quath. Bang Vat.**

Dose ½ to 2 tolas, to be taken twice a day. Chief ingredients are Trivrit, Vidari and Kokilaksha. Demulcent, diuretic, tonic and purgative. Useful in gout, gonorrhœa, haematuria, obesity, orchitis and gravel.

**Dashamool Quath.**

Sha. M. Ch. 2. V. 31.

Dose ½ to 2 tolas, to be taken twice a day. Ingredients are Shaliparni, Frastiparni, Brihati, Kantakarika, Gokshuraka, Bilwa, Agnimantha, Shyonaka, Kashmari and Patala. Alterative, bitter tonic. Extensively used in fevers and puerperal diseases, *e.g.* cough, cold, neuralgia, giddiness, headache, etc.

**Dadimatwak Quath.**

Dose ½ to 2 tolas, to be taken thrice a day Astringent, alterative. Useful in bowel complaints diarrhœa, dysentery, etc

No. 134. **Dadimamooltwak Quath.**

Dose ½ to 2 tolas, to be taken in the morning. Mainly used to expel tape worm.

**Darvyadi Quath.**

Sha M. Ch. 2.

Dose ½ to 1 tola, to be taken twice a day. Chief ingredients are Darvi, Rasanjana, Musta, Bhallataka, Bilva, Kirata, Vasa, &c. Bitter tonic, antiperiodic, astringent and stimulant. Recommended in Shastras for leucorrhœa, menorrhagia and other diseases of genito-urinary system. Removes headache, anorexia, restlessness, dullness and such other accompaniments of leucorrhœa.

## QUATHS.

### Devdarvadi Quath.

Sha. M. Ch. 2.

Dose ½ to 2 tolas. Chief ingredients are Devdar, Vacha, Kustha, Pippali, Shunthi, Katphala, Kirata, Katuki, Brihati, Gudoochi, Gokshuraka, Shringi, etc. Bitter tonic, alterative, stimulant. Recommended in Shastras for after-pains and other after-labour troubles, as colic, fever, headache, etc. It is generally given to women in confinement as a prophilactic means.

### Nimbadi Quath. Bhav. Masu.

Dose ½ to 2 tolas, to be taken twice a day. Chief ingredients are Nimba, Parpat, Patha, Katuki, Haritaki, Vasa, Valaka, Dhanvayasa, etc. Bitter tonic, anti-periodic, aperient. Recommended in jaundice, worms, hepatitis, leprosy, etc.

### Nyagrodhadigana Quath.

S. Su. Ch. 38.

Chief ingredients are Panchvalkala, Madhuka, Lodhra, Bhallatak and other astringent barks. Astringent. Useful for washing in ulcers.

### Panchvalkal Quath.

Chief ingredients are Aswattha, Pippala, Udambara, Nichula. Astringent. Useful for washing in pruritus valve, chronic tonsilitis, sinus, leucorrhœa, stomatitis.

### Patoladi Quath.

Vag. U. Ch. 22.

Dose ½ to 2 tolas, to be taken twice a day, with Swarjikakshara. Chief ingredients are Patola, Triphala, Trayamana, Katuki, Darvi, Gudoochi etc. Alterative, laxative and bitter tonic. Useful in fevers, stomatitis, dyspepsia, enlargement of the spleen or liver, jaundice, dropsy, pruritus ani, etc.

## Pathyadi Quath.

Sha. M. Ch. 2.

Dose ½ to 2 tolas, to be taken twice a day. Chief ingredients are Triphala, Kirata and Gudoochi. Alterative, bitter tonic and antiperiodic. Removes dyspepsia and feverishness. Specially suitable in hemicrania and headache etc.

## Pathadikashaya.

Ch. Sha. Ch. VIII.

Dose ½ to 2 tolas, to be taken twice a day. Chief ingredients are Patha, Deodar, Musta, Murva, Gudoochi, Kirata, Katuki, Sariva, Indrayava etc. Alterative, bitter tonic, diuretic. Specially given to purify mother's milk. Cures dyspepsia, restores lost appetite, improves general health. It is also useful in affections of genito urinary system.

## Punarnavadi Quath.

Sha. M. Ch. 2.

Dose ½ to 2 tolas, to be taken twice a day. Chief ingredients are Punarnava, Nimbatwaka, Darvi, Katuki, Shunthi, Gudoochi, Patola, etc. Bitter tonic, alterative, laxative, antiperiodic, diuretic. Useful in bubo, rheumatism (chronic) dropsy etc. Add 5 to 15 grs. Sourkshara before taking.

## Brihatyadigana Quath.

Su. Su. Ch. 38.

Dose ½ to 2 tolas, twice a day. Chief ingredients are Brihati, Kantakarika, Indrayava, Patha and Yasthimadhu Expectorant, demulcent, diuretic, tonic. Useful in cough, asthma, bronchitis and other chest affections. It is also useful in cystitis, dysuria, incontinence of urine and other genito-urinary affections.

## Manjisthadi Quath. (Laghu)

Sha. M. Ch. II.

Dose ½ to 2 tolas, to be taken twice a day. Chief

ingredients are Manjishtha, Triphala, Katuki, Vacha, Darvi, Gudoochi, Nimbatwak. Alterative, diuretic, astringent, antiperiodic, tonic, stimulant. Recognised as a blood purifier. Improves general health, and is useful in acne, scrofula, boils, leprosy, and other skin diseases due to impure blood.

### Manjisthadi Quath. (Brihat)

Sha. M. Ch. II.

Dose ½ to 2 tolas, to be taken twice a day. Chief ingredients are Manjistha, Musta, Kutajatwak, Gudoochi, Darvi, Nimbatwak, Moorva, Sariva etc. In all contains 45 drugs. Alterative, bitter tonic. Uses same as above.

### Mundi Quath.

Dose ½ to 2 tolas, to be taken twice a day. Alterative, demulcent. Useful as an alterative in syphilis, boils, rheumatism and ulcers; as a demulcent, in urethritis.

### Mutravirechana Quath.

Ch. Su. Ch. IV.

Dose ½ to 2 tolas, twice a day. Chief ingredients are Gokshuraka, Arka, Apamarga. Ashmabheda, Darbha and Kokilaksha. Diuretic, demulcent, tonic. Very useful in all diseases of genito-urinary tract. Gives good results in enlargement of the prostrate gland, rheumatism, dysuria, cystitis, gonorrhœa, gleet, &c. Increases flow of urine and allays irritation of the mucus membrane of genito-urinary system.

### Mootrasangrahana Quath.

Ch. Su. Ch. IV.

Dose ½ to 2 tolas, twice a day. Chief ingredients are Jambu-asthi, Amrasthi, Ashwatthatwak, Karpuratwak and Bhallatak. Astringent, alterative, tonic. Specially useful in diabetes insipidus.

**Rasnadi Quath.**

Sha M. Ch. II.

Dose ½ to 2 tolas, to be taken twice a day. Chief ingredients are Rasna, Gudoochi, Devdara, Gokshuraka, Punarnava. Bitter tonic, aperient, diuretic. Useful in rheumatism, paraplegia, sciatica, hemiplegia, lumbago and other nervous diseases.

**Rasnadi Quath. (Maha)**

Sha. M. Ch. II.

Dose ½ to 2 tolas, to be taken twice a day. Chief ingredients are Rasna, Dhanvayasa, Devdara, Shathi, Vacha, Vasa, Shunthi, Chavya, Punarnava, Shatavari, etc. Uses same as above.

**Vachadigana Quath.**

S. Su. Ch. 38

Dose ½ to 2 tolas to be taken twice a day. Chief ingredients are Vacha, Musta, Vishaa, Devdara, Nagapushpa etc. Tonic and alterative; employed to purify mother's milk.

**Varoona Quath.**

Dose ½ to 2 tolas, to be taken twice a day. Stomachic, tonic, laxative, diuretic. Promotes appetite and increases the secretion of bile. This is used in dropsy, urinary disorders and incalculus affections, as a diuretic. As an alterative, it is very much used in chronic enlargements of glands, as liver and spleen; and in boils, abscesses, ulcers etc. It is also useful in affections of bladder and uterus.

**Varoonadi Quath.**

Yoga-Ashmari.

Dose ½ to 2 tolas, to be taken with Yavakshara three times a day. Varuna and Gokshuraka are the sole ingredients. Diuretic, demulcent. Useful in dysuria, enlargement of prostrate gland, gonorrhœa, chyluria, rheumatism. As an alterative in abscesses, ulcers, etc.

**Vidarigandhadigana Quath**

S. Su. Ch. 38.

Dose ½ to 2 tolas, to be taken twice a day. Chief ingredients are Shaliparni, Vidari, Gokshuraka, Shatavari, Sariva, Punarnava, Brihati, etc. Bitter tonic, nutritive, expectorant, alterative and diuretic. Reduces temperature, promotes appetite cures cough, gives tone and nutrition to the body and is specially suitable for phthysis.

**Virtarvadi Quath.**

S. Su. Ch. 38.

Dose ½ to 2 tolas to be given twice a day. Chief ingredients are Virataru, Darbha, Ashmabheda, Arka, Vasa, Apamarga, Gokshuraka etc. Diuretic, demulcent. Useful in calculi gravel, dysuria, gonorrhœa and uric acid diathesis and other urinary disorders; also in rheumatic affections.

**Shathyadi Quath.**

Ch. Chi. Ch. III.

Dose ½ to 2 tolas, to be taken twice a day. Chief ingredients are Shathi, Kustha. Kantakarika. Shringi, Gudoochi, Patha, Kirata etc. Stimulant, alterative, bitter tonic, expectorant. Cures dyspepsia. Useful in giddiness and hysteria; also in bronchial affections.

**Sharpunkha Quath.**

Dose ½ to 2 tolas, to be taken twice a day. Alterative, tonic, diuretic. Useful in cough, derangement of the liver, spleen and kidneys and in gonorrhœa.

**Saptaparna Quath.**

Dose ½ to 2 tolas, to be taken twice a day. Bitter tonic, anthelmintic and antiperiodic. Useful in malarial fever. Unlike quinine, it has no bad after effects. Also useful in dyspepsia and chronic diarrhœa.

### Sariva (shwet) Quath.

Dose ½ to 2 tolas, to be taken twice a day. Valuable alterative, diaphoretic, diuretic and tonic. Useful as a diuretic in rheumatic pains, boils, scanty and high coloured urine, gravel etc. As a diaphoretic and tonic, it is given in fevers with loss of appetite and disinclination for food. As an alterative, it is valuable in chronic rheumatism, skin diseases, scrofula, syphilis, cachexia, constitutional debility, etc.

### Surasadigana Quath.

S. Su. Ch. 38.

Chief ingredients are Surasa, Rohisha, Kshawaka, Katphala, Nirgundi, etc. Antiseptic. Useful as an antiseptic wash in ulcers.

### Haridradi Quath.

S. Su. Ch. 38.

Dose ½ to 2 tolas, to be taken twice a day. Chief ingredients are Darvi, Indrayava, Yasthimadhu,etc. Tonic, antiperiodic. Purifies mother's milk: also cures chyluria and other diseases of urinary tract.

## CHOORNA (Powder Mixtures.)

**General directions.**—Usually the powders are taken with either milk or water. Where no direction be given, water is the only **Anupan.**

Those who dislike powders, should order out special tablets of them (which we make to order), or should prepare an infusion of the same, the process being the same as that of preparing tea.

The powders are sometimes taken with Ghrita, honey, sugar; the proportion of these should be just sufficient to mix the dose.

Wherever the **Anupan** is Ghrita or honey with milk, the dose should be first mixed with Ghrita or honey, and milk to be taken thereafter.

We sell powder mixtures in packed bottles only. The following prices are for ¼ lb. bottles only. Larger sizes can be had at proportionately cheaper prices.

---

### Amrita.

Dose 20 to 40 grs., to be taken twice a day with water. Bitter tonic, stomachic, diuretic, alterative, and antiperiodic. Useful as a remedy for dyspepsia, malaria, atonic diarrhœa; leucorrhœa, menorrhagia, and other female complaints.

### Arka-mool Churna.

Dose, as a tonic 3 to 10 grs.; as an emetic 30 to 60 grs., to be given with warm water when required as an emetic. As a tonic, to be taken three times a day. Alterative, intestinal tonic, emetic. For dysentery, this is a specific; also useful in cough, hoarseness, bronchitis, asthma and other chest affections. Best substitute for Ipecac (*Vide* Indigenous Drugs Committee Report).

**Avalgujadi Lepa.**

Ni. Part III.

Directions for use: Paste of the powder with lemon juice or whey should be applied on the part affected. Chief ingredients are Bakuchi seeds and Chakramarda seeds. Very largely used in ringworm and eczema; and pityrisis, psoriasis and other skin diseases.

**Ashwagandha Churna.**

Dose 20 to 40 grs., to be taken twice a day with milk. Tonic. Alterative. Useful in sexual and general debility; rheumatism, old age; consumption, emaciation of children and nervous diseases. It is also used in leucorrhœa.

**Ashwagandhadi Churna.**

Sha. M. Ch. VI.

Dose 20 to 80 grs., to be taken twice a day with milk. The only two ingredients are Ashwagandha and Vriddhadarak. Alterative, tonic. Removes sexual debility, spermatorrhœa and other conditions of debility, such as, of old age, leucorrhœa, etc.

**Eladi Churna.** Bhav. mutra

Dose 10 to 40 grs., to be taken three times a day with rice water. Chief ingredients are Ela, Ashmabheda, Pippali, Trapusha, and Shilajatu. Diuretic and demulcent. Very useful in dysuria, incontinence of urine and like affections of urinary tract. It is also useful in gout. In acute or inflammatory gonorrhœa there is no better remedy, as it renders the urine alkaline and unirritating. In bronchitis and pneumonia, it renders the secretion less tenacious. It gives good results in influenza also.

**Kakubhadi Churna.** Bhai.

Dose 10 to 40 grs., to be taken in the morning

with ghrita. Chief ingredients are Kakubha, Vacha, Rasna, Shathi, Kusha, Gangaruki, etc. Tonic, stimulant, alterative. Useful in Angina pectoris (between attacks) and other heart diseases.

**Katu Rohini.**

Dose 10 to 15 grs., to be taken thrice a day with milk; or with Swarjikakshar in dyspepsia and with Navasagar in liver complaints. Bread should be avoided in diet. Tonic, antiperiodic, aperient. Very good remedy in dyspepsia, bilious fever, liver complaints and jaundice. This is a valuable antiperiodic in low continued fevers; also given to children in worms.

**Kanduprashaman Churna.**

Cha. Su. Ch. IV.

To be dusted over the affected part after thoroughly washing with Snanaraja. Disinfectant. Useful as a dusting powder in pruritus valve, prurigo and other itching skin affections. Chief ingredients are Chandan, Valaka, Karanja, Nimbatwak, Sarshapa, Darvi, Kutajatwak, etc.

**Kapitthapatra Churna.**

Dose 10 to 40 grs., to be taken three times a day with water. Reduces red sand, chyle from urine, and is therefore useful in uric acid diatheses, chyluria and calculi renal and other urinary and calculous affections. This drug has shown marvellous effects specially in chyluria.

**Kapitthashtak Churna.**

Sha. M. Ch. VI.

Dose 10 to 40 grs., to be taken before or with meals, with water or whey. Chief ingredients are Kapittha, Dadima, Chincha, Bilva, Dhatakipushpa, Trikatu, etc. Stomachic, stimulant. Useful in nausea, loss of appetite, diarrhœa, and other bowel complaints.

**Karpastwak.**

Dose ½ to 1 tola, to be taken three times a day with 10 grs. of cinnamom powder. Emmenagogue hæmostatic. Useful in dysmenorrhœa, uterin haemorrhage, abortion, retained placenta, etc.

**Kindaru.**

Dose 10 to 30 grs., to be taken three times a day, with Sindava, Shunthi, etc. Stimulant. This is largely used in hernia (*see* Hernia).

**Kirata Churna.**

Dose 15 to 30 grs., to be taken three times a day with water or as an infusion. Bitter tonic, stomachic, laxative and febrifuge. Useful remedy in atonic dyspepsia, indigestion ; excites appetite, strengthens digestion, diminishes flatulence, hyperacidity and biliousness.

**Kirmani.**

Dose 15 to 60 grs., to be taken on an empty stomach with warm water preceded and followed by a purgative of castor oil. It kills round worms.

**Kuberaksh.**

Dose 5 to 20 grs., to be taken with Saindhav twice a day. Alterative, tonic. Used in general debility, flatulence, worms, hernia, indigestion, etc.

**Kusthadi Lepa.**

Bhav. Kushtha.

Chief ingredients are Kustha, Vidanga, Chakramarda, etc. The paste of this powder with lemon juice or whey should be applied on the affected part. Specially useful in ringworm.

**Kustumbarvadi Lepa.**

Su. Chi. Ch. XX.

Chief ingredients are Dhanyaka, Vacha, Lodhra

and Kustha. Paste of this powder should be applied on the affected part. Useful in acne.

### Ksharadwaya Churna.

Dose 5 to 30 grs. to be taken with water. Ingredients are Yavakshara and Swarjikakshara. Antacid, diuretic and uric acid solvent; most valuable in acute rheumatism and gout. Also useful in dyspepsia, biliousness, hyperacidity, bronchitis and gonorrhœa.

### 8 (Laghu) Gangadhar Churna.

Sha. M. Ch. VI.

Dose 20 to 40 grs., to be taken three times a day with whey. Chief ingredients are Musta, Indrayava Bilva, Lodhra, Mocharasa, Dhatakipushpa. Astringent, tonic. Useful in chronic diarrhœa. It stops diarrhœa, gives tone to the intestines, promotes appetite and increases digestive power.

### (Vridhha) Gangadhar Churna.

Sha. M. Ch. VI.

Dose 20 to 40 grs., to be taken three times a day with whey. Chief ingredients are Musta, Syonaka, Shunthi, Lodhra, Dhatakipushpa, Mocharasa, Patha, Kutajatwak, Indrayava. Astringent, tonic. Use same as above.

### Gokshuraka Churna.

Dose 10 to 20 grs., to be taken thrice a day with milk or barley water. Demulcent and diuretic. A useful remedy for nocturnal seminal emissions, incontinence of urine, gonorrhœa, gleet and sexual debility.

### Gokshurakadi Churna.

Dose 10 to 30 grs., to be taken three times a day with milk or barley water. Only ingredients are Gokshuraka and Kokilaksha. Demulcent and diuretic. Useful remedy for dysuria, incontinence of urine, uric acid diatheses, gravel and catarrh of Urinary organs. Also useful in spermatorrhœa and other seminal affections.

**Chandanadi Kalka.**

Ch. Chi. Ch. 23.

Dose 20 to 80 grs. To be taken 1½ hours after meals with barley water. Chief ingredients are Chandana, Draksha, Mansi, Valaka, etc. Stimulant, disinfectant and demulcent. Useful in vomiting, acute and sub-acute gonorrhœa, cystitis, and other genito urinary affections.

**Chandrodaya Anupan.** Bhai.

Dose 4 to 12 grs., to be taken with Chandrodayarasa. Chief ingredients are Vanshalochana, Trikatu, Musk. Tonic, stimulant and expectorant. Useful in cough, phthisis, general debility, sexual debility, &c.

**Chitraka.**

Dose 10 to 30 grs., to be taken before meals. Alterative, gastric stimulant. Useful in chronic diarrhœa, dyspepsia and general anasarca.

**Chitrakmuladi Churna.**

Dose 10 to 30 grs., to be taken three times a day with water. Chief ingredients are Chitraka, Brahmi and Vacha. Alterative, stimulant, tonic and diuretic. Useful in epilepsy, hysteria, mania and other mental disorders.

**Dusting Powder.**

Useful in lichen and other skin affections.

No. 915. **Chopchinyadi Churna.**

Ni. Part III.

Dose ¼ to 1 tola, to be taken with milk twice

a day. Chief ingredients are Chopchini, sugar, Pippali, Pippalimoola, Maricha, Lavanga, Akarkarabha, Parasikayavani, Vidang, etc. Alterative, stimulant, diaphoretic and sedative. Useful in rheumatism, gout, epilepsy, general cachexia, scrofula and seminal weakness. In constitutional tertiary syphilis, this gives good results if continued for a long time.

### Chowsasthi Pippali.

Dose 6 to 24 grs., to be taken with honey and milk in the morning. Stimulant, carminative, laxative and alterative. Useful in chronic cough and other chest affections, dyspepsia, enlargement of the spleen, &c.

### Jatiphaladi Churna.

Sha. M. Ch. VI.

Dose 12 to 24 grs., to be taken with honey twice a day. 12 grs. of this mixture contains 3 grs. of Vijaya (Canabis Indica). Chief ingredients are Vijaya, Jatiphala, Karpura, Ela, Lawanga, Chitraka, Vanshlochana, etc. Sedative, anodyne, and antispasmodic. Useful in migraine, asthma, delirium, colic, neuralgia, cancer, pains of last stages in phthysis, acute mania, menorrhagia, dysmenorrhœa, spasmodic cough, etc., etc.

### Talisadi Churna.

Sha. M. Ch. VI.

Dose 20 to 60 grs., to be taken before meals. Chief ingredients are Talispatra, Trikatu, Vanshlochana, Kasni, Ela, sugar, &c. Stimulant, expectorant, laxative and alterative. Useful in anorexia, chronic cough and other chest affections, dyspepsia, enlargement of the spleen, etc.

### Tikta Jiraka.

Dose 20 to 60 grs., to be given on an empty stomach, followed by a purgative such as castor oil. Anthelmintic, stomachic, antiperiodic and alterative. Useful in worms, loss of appetite, dyspepsia, leucoderma, psoriasis, etc.

### Tiladi Lepa.

Su. Chi. Ch. V.

Chief ingredients are Tila, Sarshapa, Yava, Shigrutwak, Swarjika, etc. A poultice prepared with this powder should be applied on the parts affected. Specially suitable in gout.

### Triphala Churna.

Sha. M. Ch. VI.

Dose ¼ to ½ tola, to be taken with milk in the morning or at bed time. Sole ingredients are Haritaki, Bibhitaka and Amalaka. Alterative, astringent and aperient. Regulates the bowels. Largely used in dyspepsia, chronic diarrhœa, hiccough and colic. Specially beneficial in eye diseases and internal hæmorrhages.

### Trivritadi Churna.

Sha. U. Ch, IV.

Dose ½ to 1 tola, to be taken with water. Purgative, alterative and carminative. Removes constipation, indigestion and flatulence; is particularly beneficial in rheumatism and paralytic affections, melancholia, gout, dropsy, &c.

### Dashanga Lepa.

Sha. U. Ch. XI.

The paste of this lepa made with water or rose water, should be applied on the affected part. Useful in abscesses, neuralgia, erysipelas, mumps, boils, etc. Chief ingredients are Shirishatwak, Yastimadhu, Tagar, Raktachandan, Ela, Mansi, Darvi, Kustha, Valaka, etc.

## CHOORNA (Powder Mixtures.)

### Dadimastaka.

Sha. M. Ch. VI.

Dose 20 to 60 grs., to be taken before meals. Chief ingredients are Dadima, Ela, Trikatu, Trijat and sugar. Gastric stimulant and alterative. Useful in anorexia; promotes appetite and helps digestion. Also useful in diarrhœa.

### Doshaghna Lepa.

Sha. U. Ch. XI.

Chief ingredients are Punarnava, Deodara, Shunthi, Sarshapa and Shigrutwak. Rubefacient. The paste of this lepa made with whey should be applied on the affected part in thick layer. Useful in abscess, goitre, scrofula, neuralgia, bubo, etc.

### Dwiruttar Hinguadi Churna.

Ch. Chi. Ch. 10.

Dose 20 to 60 grs., to be taken twice a day with water. Chief ingredients are Hingu, Vacha, Chitraka, Kustha, Sauvarchala and Vidanga. Carminative, stimulant, alterative. Useful in tympanitis, hysteria, flatulance, etc.

### Dhanyak Churna.

Dose 10 to 40 grs., to be taken with sodium cloride (salt). Aromatic, stomachic, stimulant, carminative. Useful in vomiting, dyspepsia, common catarrh, and as a gargle in stomatitis. It is much used as a flavouring agent and as a corrective to griping medicines.

### Nagapushpa.

Dose 6 to 24 grs., to be taken with butter three times a day. Bitter, aromatic, and sudorific. Useful in dysentery.

### Narsinha Churna.

Vag. Chi. Ch. 19.

Dose 10 to 40 grs., to be taken twice a day with

ghee and sugar. Chief ingredients are Triphala, Trikatu, Tila, and Bhallataka. Stimulant, tonic, alterative. Useful in sexual debility, alcoholism, leprosy, neuralgia and dyspepsia. This is also used in syphilis. Capsicum and other pungent spices and oils and heat to be avoided.

### Panchasama Churna.

Sha. M. Ch. VI.

Dose 20 to 80 grs., to be taken with water. Chief ingredients are Shunthi, Haritaki, Pippali, Trivrit and Krishnalavana. Purgative, stimulant, carminative. Useful in indigestion, tympanitis, colic and other intestinal disorders. Also beneficial in rheumatic and paralytic affections, melancholia, gout, dropsy, etc.

### Parpat Churna.

Dose ½ to 1 tola, to be taken every three hours with water of Dhanyak and Grapes. Bitter tonic and antiperiodic. Useful in fevers of all kinds, specially suitable in fevers with gastric irritation and nervous depression. In fevers, it allays thirst, reduces dryness of the throat and stops vomiting, relieves the burning sensation of hands and feet. It is also useful in headache and intestinal hæmorrhage.

### Parsikayavani.

Dose 4 to 12 grs., to be taken three times a day or whenever necessary. Sedative, antispasmodic, anodyne. Useful in enlargement of prostrate gland, paralysis agitans, insomnia, acute mania, asthma, convulsions of children, delirium tremens, colic.

### Pippalimool.

Dose 6 to 24 grs., to be taken three times a day with molasses. Stimulant, carminative, alterative. Useful in chest affections, dyspepsia, chronic cough, enlargement of the spleen, and other abdominal viscera, gout, lumbago, etc. Also prescribed by physicians in insomnia.

### 9 Pippalyadi Churna.

Ch. Chi. Ch. 19.

Dose 15 to 90 grs., to be taken three times a day with water. Chief ingredients are Pippali, Patha, Sariva, Brihati, Chitraka, 5 salts and Yavakkshara, etc. Alterative, tonic, antacid, antilithic, diuretic. Useful in after pains, rheumatism, gout, acute gonorrhœa, dyspepsia, sprue, influenza. dysuria, gravel, uric acid diathesis, etc.

### Pippalyadi-Pratisaran. Vag.

To be rubbed on the teeth and gums. The only ingredients are Pippali, Amalaka and Dhatakipushpa. Recommended in Shastras for toothache.

### Peenashari-Tamaku.

Chief ingredients are Karpura, Boric acid and Tobacco. Useful as snuff in cold and ozœna.

### Punarnava.

Dose 20 to 60 grs., to be taken three times a day. Stomachic, laxative, diuretic and expectorant. Useful in dropsy, jaundice, enlargement of liver and spleen, ascites, anasarca, scanty urine, gonorrhœa. It is also used in asthma.

### Pushyanuga Churna.

Ch. Chi. Ch. 3

Dose 20 to 60 grs. to be taken twice a day with rice water. Chief ingredients are Patha, Jambuasthi, Amrasthi, Ashmabheda, Kutajatwak, Lodhra, Bilvapeshika, Dhatakipushpa, etc. Alterative, tonic, astringent, diuretic. Useful in leucorrhœa, menorrhagia and other women complaints.

**Bidalak Lepa.**

Sha. U. Ch. 13.

The paste of this lepa made with water or rose water should be applied to the outside of the affected eye. Chief ingredients are Gairika, Rasanjana, Madhuka and Saindhava. Useful in conjunctivitis and other eye diseases.

**Bhaskar Lavan Churna.**

Sha. M. Ch. 6.

Dose 20 to 60 grs., to be taken before or with food Chief ingredients are Saindhava, Bida, Sauvarchala, Dhanyaka, Pippali, Pippalimoola, Amlavetasa, etc. Gastric stimulant, carminative. Useful in indigestion, flatulence, nausea, costiveness, loss of appetite and other bowel complaints.

**Bhoonimbadi Churna.**

Ch. Chi. Ch. 19.

Dose 20 to 60 grs., to be taken three times a day with whey. Chief ingredients are Kirata, Katuki, Trikatu, Musta, Indrayava, Chitraka and Kutajatwak. Bitter tonic, intestinal tonic, antiperiodic and gastric stimulant. Specially suitable for dyspepsia and chronic diarrhœa. Promotes appetite, helps digestion, gives tone to the intestines and stops diarrhœa. It is also useful in fevers, dysentery and worms. Also in internal hæmorrhages, chronic chest diseases as asthma and renal colic. Also given in cholera to arrest vomiting.

**Manjisthadi Lepa.**

S. Chi. Ch. 18.

Chief ingredients are Manjistha, Gudoochi, Shigru, Punarnava, Arka, Kustha, Lodhra. The paste of this lepa should be applied on the affected part. Useful in boils, erysipelas, goitre, abscess, etc.

No. 8 **Madanadivaman.**

Dose as an expectorant 5 to 15 grs., as an emetic 20 to 60 grs. to be taken with tepid water. Ingredients are Madanphala, Arkamoola and Yasthimadhu. Expectorant, demulcent and emetic. Useful as an expectorant in bronchitis and other chest affections; and as an emetic in croup, colic, headache, orchitis, indigestion, poisonous effects.

**Musalyadi Churna.**

Sha. M. Ch. 6.

Dose 20 to 60 grs., to be taken twice a day with milk. Chief ingredients are Moosali, Gokshuraka, Shalmalimoola, Vanari and Gudoochi-satva. Tonic nutritive, alterative and aphrodisiac. Very valuable in sexual debility. Also useful in leucorrhœa, menstrual derangements due to general debility and paralysis.

**Medhya Rasayana.**

Ch. Chi. Ch. 1.

Dose 20 to 60 grs., to be taken three times a day with milk. Chief ingredients are Brahmi, Shankhpushpi, Gudoochi, and Yastimadhu. Alterative, demulcent, diuretic, stimulant, tonic. Useful in insomnia, hoarseness, mania, epilepsy, as also cough, bronchitis and other chest affections.

**Yavanikhandav Churna.**

Sha. M. Ch. VI.

Dose 20 to 60 grs., to be taken twice a day before or with food. Chief ingredients are Yavani, Dadima seeds, Shunthi, Chincha, Amlavetasa, Krishnalavana, Jiraka, Sugar, &c. Gastric stimulant, carminative. Useful in indigestion, loss of appetite, dyspepsia, etc.

### Yastimadhu Churna.

Dose 20 to 60 grs., to be taken three times a day with honey. Demulcent, expectorant, slightly laxative. Useful in inflammatory affections, catarrh, cough, hoarseness, asthma, laryngitis, bronchitis, and gonorrhœa.

### Rasayana Churna.

Vag. U. Ch. 39.

Dose 20 to 60 grs. to be taken twice a day with Ghee and sugar followed by milk. Chief ingredients are Gudoochi, Gokshuraka and Amalaka. Bitter tonic, demulcent, alterative, diuretic. Eliminates waste, promotes appetite, improves general health and removes disorders of digestive and urinary organs—hence it gives good results in general debility and sexual debility due to disorders of the digestive or urinary organs.

### Pulv. Rhei Radix (Revanchi twak).

Dose 3 to 10 grs., for repeated doses, and 15 to 30 grs. for a single dose. Aperient, stomachic, tonic and astringent. Stimulates the muscular layer of the bowels and the intestinal glands. Is useful in atonic dyspepsia and urticaria. It may be used with advantage in diarrhœa, due to irritating substances in the intestines.

### Rohitak Churna.

Dose 20 to 60 grs., to be taken three times a day with water. Alterative, astringent, tonic. Has special effect on liver and spleen. Useful in hepatitis, enlargement of spleen, general debility and scrofula.

### Lavangadya Churna.

Sha. M. Ch. 6.

Dose 20 to 60 grs., to be taken three times a day with water. Chief ingredients are Lavanga, Karpura, Kankola Jatiphala, sugar, &c. Sedative, antispasmodic, carminative, expectorant, diaphoretic, antiseptic. Useful in cold, hiccough, diarrhœa, lumbago, whooping cough, flatulence and urinary affections.

### Lodhradi Churna.

Ch. Chi. Ch. 15.

Chief ingredients are Lodhra, Katphala, Lajjalu and Dhatakipushpa. Astringent. Recommended for local use as dusting powder in ulcers.

### Vacha Churna.

Dose 20 to 40 grs., to be taken three times a day. Bitter, stimulant, tonic, carminative. Useful in ague, habitual constipation, atonic dyspepsia, colic, flatulence. Also used in epilepsy, mania and other mental disorders.

### Vachadi Lepa. S. Chi. Ch. 20.

The paste of this lepa should be applied on the affected part. Chief ingredients are Vacha, Sarshapa and Darvi. Useful for local application in acne and boils.

### Vadavanal Churna.

Sha. M. Ch. VI.

Dose 10 to 40 grs., to be taken twice a day with water. Chief ingredients are Saindhava, Pippalimoola, Pippali, Chitraka, Shunthi and Haritaki. Stimulant, aperient, alterative, expectorant and tonic. Useful in dyspepsia, indigestion, loss of appetite, cough and other intestinal and chest affections.

### Vidang Churna.

Dose 60 to 240 grs., to be taken on an empty stomach preceded on the last night by a purgative and followed by a purgative as castor oil after 3 or 4 hours. For worms and for skin diseases to be taken in the morning with water, followed after six hours, by simple diet of mung water and rice. Stimulant, alterative, anthelmintic, carminative. Specific for tape worm. Is also used in flatulence and dyspepsia as a carminative and in skin diseases and rheumatism as an alterative.

**Vidangtandul Prayoga.**

S. Chi. Ch. 27.

Dose ½ to 1 tola, to be taken in the morning with water, mung water and rice only. Diet should be without salt and with Amalak and Ghrit. Ingredients are Vidang and Yashthimadhu. This prayoga should be continued at least for a month. Alterative: reduces obesity and chyluria. It has often cured leprosy. Vidangtandul Churna without the dietetic restrictions may be given in worms instead of simple Vidang Churna.

**Vidangadi Churna.** Bhav.

Dose ½ to 1 tola, to be taken on an empty stomach, preceded overnight by a light purge. Chief ingredients are Vidanga, Yastimadhu, Trikatu, Dantimoola, Trivrit and Chitraka. Anthelmintic, stimulant, alterative and purgative. Useful in tape worms, dyspepsia, flatulence, etc.

**Vishadi Churna.** Vag.

Dose 1 to 4 grs. for children to be taken three times a day with honey. Sole ingredients are Visha, Shringi, Pippali and Yastimadhu. Demulcent, expectorant, alterative. Specially suitable for cold and other diseases of children.

**Vaishvanar Churna.** Gada.

Dose 20 to 60 grs. to be taken twice a day with Swarjikakshar. Chief ingredients are Saindhava, Ajmoda, Yavani, Pippali, Shunthi and Haritaki. Gastric stimulant, aperient, carminative. Useful in indigestion, dyspepsia, tympânitis, flatulence, acid eructations, heart-burn, colic, hysteria, etc.

## CHOORNA (Powder Mixtures.)

### Shakrayava Churna.

Dose: 20 to 60 grs., three times a day with sugar. Antiperiodic, tonic, astringent. It gives strength to the intestinal walls. Useful in fever, chronic diarrhœa, dysentery, internal hæmorrhages, worms (specially of children), chronic chest diseases, etc.

### Shatavaryadi Churna.

Sha. M. Ch. 6.

Dose : 20 to 60 grs. to be taken twice a day with milk. Chief ingredients are Shatavari, Gokshuraka, Gangeruki, Atibala and Kokilaksha. Nutritive, tonic and demulcent. Specially useful in sexual debility.

### Shirovirechan Churna.

Chief ingredients are Katphalatwak and Vidanga. Sternutatory : useful as snuff in fainting.

### Shiladi Churna. S. U. Ch. 14.

Chief ingredients are Manashila, Ela, Tagara and Saindhava. Recommended in Shastras for local application in stye.

### Shiva Churna.

Dose : 30 to 120 grs. Purgative, astringent, alterative. Beneficial in indigestion, diarrhœa, dysentery and such other gastric disorders.

### Shukrashodhan Churna.

Ch. S. Ch. 4.

Dose : ¼ to 1 tola, to be taken twice a day with honey or ghee and sugar, followed by milk. Chief ingredients are Kustha, Samudraphena, Kokilaksha, Katphala, etc. Diuretic, stimulant, astringent. Specially useful in spermatorrhœa and other seminal affections.

**Shringyadi Churna** (Infant Powder).

Sha. M. Ch. 6.

Dose: 1 to 4 grs., to be given three times a day with honey. Sole ingredients are Shringi, Visha and Pippali. Gastric stimulant, bitter astringent, alterative. Beneficial in cough, diarrhœa (infantile,) bronchitis, teething, incontinence of urine and other diseases of children.

**Shireeshadi Lepa.**

S. Ka. Ch. 6.

Chief ingredients are Shirishatwak, Ajmoda, Yavani, Shunthi, Pippali, etc. Recommended for local application in Bites.

**Shad-dharan Yoga.**

S. Chi. Ch. 4.

Dose: 20 to 60 grs. to be taken with Swarjika three times a day Chief ingredients are Chitraka, Indrayava, Katuki, Patha and Haritaki. Tonic, laxative, alterative. Efficacious in atonic dyspepsia and other intestinal disorders.

**Saptamrit.** R. Chin.

Dose: 12 to 24 grs., to be taken at night with Ghee and sugar, followed by milk for 21 days. Chief ingredients are Triphala, Loha Bhasma and Yastimadhu. Alterative, tonic, hœmatinic. Recommended in Shastras for eye diseases, headache, hemicrania, epistaxis, aphonia, etc. Heavy meals at night should be avoided—if possible, no other food except milk should be taken.

. **Samudrafen** (Cuttlefish bone)

Useful as a dusting powder in otorrhœa.

No. 898. **Sarshapadi Lepa.** Bhav.

Chief ingredients are Sarshapa, Shanabija, Yava, and Moolakabija. Useful for local application in goitre, scrofula, abscesses, boils and other local inflammations. This lepa should be prepared in a poultice and should be applied on the affected part.

**Samudraka-virechan Churna.** Rs. 0 12 0

Dose: 60 to 120 grs. in repeated doses; ½ to 1 oz. for a single dose. Chief ingredients are Sodium Sulphate, Sodium-bicarbonate, &c. Purgative. Efficacious in indigestion, constipation, vomiting, headache, colic, nephritis, stomatitis, nausea, facial paralysis, and all other diseases where a good purgative is required.

**Saraswat Churna.** Bhav.

Dose: 20 to 80 grs., to be taken three times a day with milk. Chief ingredients are Kustha, Aswagandha, Saindhava, Ajmoda, Jiraka, Trikatu, Patha, Shankhapushpi and Vacha. Alterative, stimulant, brain tonic. Useful in epilepsy, mania, paralysis (general,) hemiplegia, mental weakness and hoarseness of voice.

**Sitopaladi Churna.**

Sha. M. Ch. 6

Dose: 20 to 60 grs., to be taken three times a day with honey. Sole ingredients are Twak, Ela, Pippali Vanshrochana and sugar. Expectorant, stimulant. Recommended in cough, bronchitis, phthisis, chest affections, burning of the feet, &c.

**(Laghu) Sudarshan Churna***

Yogratna Samuchchaya. Dose: ½ to 1 tola, to be taken twice a day. Chief ingredients are Gudoochi, Pippalimoola, Pippali, Katuki, Abhaya, Kirata, Nimbatwak, &c. Bitter tonic. Useful in dyspepsia, dyspeptic loss of appetite, jaundice, acidity, heartburn, fever.

---

* To make infusion: keep ½ tola Sudarshan in 4 tolas of boiling water for 15 minutes, then strain. To be administered before it cools down.

### (Brihat) Sudarshana Churna *

Sha. M. Ch. 6.

Dose : ¼ to 1 tola, to be taken three times a day. Chief ingredients are Kirata and 52 other bitter tonics. Bitter tonic. Extensively used in fevers, dyspepsia, nausea.

### Snanaraj—bath powder.

The powder should be rubbed over the whole body just before bathing. Chief ingredients are Chandana, Valaka, Amalaka, etc. Aromatic, antiseptic, Useful as a bath powder in prurigo, fœtid perspiration, lichen, etc.

### Swadishta Virechan Churna.

Dose : 60 to 120 grs. to be taken at bed time. Sole ingredients are Yasthimadhu, Shatapushpi, Markandi, Gandhaka and Sugar. Purgative, demulcent. Efficacious in piles, prolapsus ani, constipation, fissure of the anus, pruritus ani. Best remedy for piles.

### Hinguadi Churna.

Sha. M. Ch. 6

Dose : 10 to 40 grs., to be taken twice a day. Chief ingredients are Hingu, Trikatu, Jiraka, Vacha, Yavakshara, Swarjika and 5 other salts. Carminative, stimulant, recommended in Shastras for nausea, hiccough, indigestion, dyspepsia, biliousness, hyperacidity, vomiting, tympanitis, colic, etc.

### Hinguashtak Churna.

Vag. Chi. Ch. 14

Dose : 20 to 60 grs., to be taken before or with food. Chief ingredients are Trikatu Ajmoda, Saindhava, Jiraka, Krishnajirak and Hingu. Gastric stimulant ; Carminative. Very popular and extensively used as a remedy for loss of appetite, indigestion, colic, dyspepsia, tympanitis, etc.

---

* See footnote on page 115.

# PILLS

We manufacture pills of one to six grains weight, just suitable to the proportion of the dose. Generally, we have given the dose as 1 to 4 pills, but it absolutely rests with the physician to determine the actual dose according to the nature of the disease.

The proportion of poison mixed in each pill, has been accurately mentioned, to enable the prescriber to fix his dose. So also is mentioned the Bhasmas occurring in the several preparations. Those preparations that contain mercury in any form are classed under the head of **Rasayanas.**

**Anupan** varies with the medicine; and we have tried to give several. Water is the only Anupan where none is mentioned.

The weight of each pill (excluding the coating material, in case of coated pills) is noted against its name, as so many grains.

### Amrita-guggula.

Asht. U. Ch. 28.

Dose: 1 to 4 pills three times a day with water or Manjisthadi Quath. Chief ingredients are Gudoochi, Ela, Vidanga, Indrayava, Triphala, Guggulu, etc. Alterative, astringent and tonic. Recommended in Shastras for rheumatism, scrofulous affections, gout, obesity, boils, ulcers, etc.

### Akarkarbhadi Gutika.

Sha M. Ch. 6.

Dose 1 to 3 pills. Each pill contains 1-3 gr. opium. Chief ingredients are opium, Akarkarabha, Kankola, Pippali, Jatiphala, Lavanga, saffron, &c. Anodyne, vascular and nervine stimulant. Efficacious in convulsions, insomnia, cough, neuralgia, after pains, alcoholism, cancer, cystitis, gout, hæmorrhages, retention of urine.

**Updanshahara. No. 1 (Cure for syphilis)**

**3 grs.**

Dose: 1 to 4 pills. Each pill contains 1-64 grs. mercuric chloride. To be taken twice a day. Sole ingredients are Mercuric chloride, Potassium Iodide, Lavanga, Kumkuma (Saffron) and Gudoochi extract. Antiseptic. Specific for syphilis. This drug should be continued for several months in cases of secondary syphilis.

**Updanshahar Gutika, No. 2.**

**3 grs.**

Dose: 1 to 4 pills twice a day after meals. Each pill contains 1-60 gr. arsenic and 1-2 gr. nux-vomica. Sole ingredients are arsenic, nux-vomica, iron and Gudoochi-rasakriya. This should be given instead of No. 1 every other week. These Nos. 1 and 2 given alternately for a long time, are an effective remedy in all stages of chancre and in cases of secondary and tertiary syphilis.

**Eliyakadi Guti.**

Dose: 1 to 4 pills, to be taken at night to be followed the next morning by Samudraka Virechan Churna. Hydragogue cathartic. Sole ingredients are Elayaka (aloes) Revanchitwak (Rhubarb root) and Katuki. Hepatic stimulant, tonic, antiperiodic. Useful in jaundice, hepatic, colic congestion of liver, hepatitis, cyrrhosis, dropsy, headache, etc. Contra indicated in pregnancy and piles.

**Eliadi Pills.**

Dose: 1 to 4 pills. Sole ingredients are aloes and myrrh. Cathartic, hepatic stimulant and emmenagogue. Useful in amenorrhœa with constipation. Contra indicated in pregnancy or piles.

**Kankayan Gutika.**

Sha. M. Ch. 7.

Dose: 1 to 4 pills. Chief ingredients are Yavani,

Hingu, Yavakshara, Swarjika, 5 salts, Trivrit, Dantimoola, Shiva, Vidanga, Chitraka and Amlavetasa. Gastric stimulant, carminative and laxative. Useful in flatulence, colic, dyspepsia, etc.

### Kanchnar Guggula.

Sha. M. Ch. 7.

Dose 1 to 4 to be taken three times a day with water or Mundi Quath or Manjisthadi Quath. Chief ingredients are Kanchnartwak, Triphala, Trikatu, Varuna and Guggulu. Alterative, tonic. Has special effect on scrofula. Useful in sinus, fistula, leprosy, ulcers, etc.

### Kasisadi Gutika.

Dose: 1 to 4, to be taken twice a day after food. Chief ingredients are Eliyaka (aloes) and Kasisa (Ferrous Sulphate). Tonic and cathartic, emmanagogue. Specific for anæmic amenorrhœa, chlorosis. Is also very valuable in Bright's disease, heart affections and scrofula. Contra indicated in pregnancy and nursing stage..

### Kishor Guggulu.

Sha. M. Ch. 7

Dose: 1 to 4 pills, three time a day with Manjisthadi Quath. Chief ingredients are Triphala, Gudoochi and Guggulu. Alterative tonic. Useful in scrofula, ulcers, boils, chronic otorrhœa, fistula, sciatica, etc. Much used in cases of rheumatism.

### Khadiradi Gutika.

Ch. Chi. Ch. 26.

To be kept into the mouth and allowed to be slowly dissolved. No more than 24 pills to be taken during 24 hours. Chief ingredients are Khadirarasa, Arimeda, Lavanga, Kankola, Jatiphala, Jatipatri and Karpura. Astringent, anæsthetic and antiseptic. Cures stomatitis, removes fœtid odour from the mouth, relieves toothache and other diseases of teeth. These pills are generally useful in diseases of mouth, throat and teeth. They remove hoarseness.

## Gokshuradi Guggulu.

Sha. M. Ch. 7.

Dose: 1 to 4 pills three times a day. Chief ingredients are Gokshuraka, Guggulu, Trikatu and Triphala. Demulcent, diuretic, alterative and tonic. Useful in albuminaria, phosphaturia, euresis, dysuria, calculi, gonorrhœa and rheumatism. It is generally useful in urinary and calculus affections.

## Chandraprabha Gutika.

Sha. M. Ch. 7.

Dose: 1 to 4 pills three times a day with milk or water. Chief ingredients are Guggulu. Trivrit, Dantimoola, Twak, Ela, Loha Bhasma, Sugar, Vanshalochana, Yavakshara, Swarjika, Makshika Bhasma, Shilajatu. Tonic, diuretic, diaphoretic, antacid. Most valuable remedy in albuminaria, phosphaturia, gout, gonorrhœa, calculi renal, etc. Also used in chicken-pox, herpes, lumbago, pruritus vulvæ, fevers, etc.

## Fever Pills.

Dose: 1 to 4 pills. Each pill contains 1/64 gr. arsenic, to be taken every six hours. very useful in pernicious malaria and other fevers. Also useful in eczema, psoriasis and other chronic skin diseases.

## Tonic Pills.

Dose: 1 to 4. To be taken twice after meals Sole ingredients are Quinine, Iron and Strychnine. Each pill contains 1/60 gr. Strychnine. Tonic, gastric, cardiac and general antiperiodic. Removes general and sexual debility. Most serviceable in hemiplegia, paraplegia and various local paralysis, many neurotic affections. Also useful in atonic dyspepsia and nocturnal enuresis. By stimulating the respiratory centre, it relieves the night sweats of phthisis and is often most valuable in bronchitis and pneumonia.

Contra-indicated in recent cases of paralysis, while rigidity exists, or in cerebral paralysis with continuance of head symptoms.

**Trayodashang Guggulu.**

Bhav.

Dose: 1 to 4 pills, to be taken three times a day. Chief ingredients are Babbulatwak, Ashwagandha, Shatavari, Gudoochi, Rasna, Gokshuraka, Parasikayavani and Guggulu. Demulcent, diuretic, aperient, tonic, alterative, sedative and anti-spasmodic. Useful in enlargement of prostrate gland, asthma, cystitis, incontinence of urine and all spasmodic affections. It also relieves internal neuralgic affections.

**Trikatuadi Gutika.**

Cha. Chi. Ch. 20.

Dose: 1 to 4. to be taken after meals with milk. Chief ingredients are Loha Bhasma, Trikatu, Triphala, Chitraka, Musta, Vidanga. Tonic alterative. Very valuable in scrofula, phthisis, anæmia, dropsy, spermatorrhœa, diabetes, general debility, sexual debility.

**Triphala Guggulu.**

Sha. M. Ch. 7.

Dose: 1 to 4 pills, to be taken three times a day with Varuna Quath. Chief ingredients are Triphala, Guggula, and Pippali. Is used in boils, carbuncle, abscesses, ulcers, sinus, fistula, etc.

**Dashang Abhrak.**

Rasa Hradaya. Rs. 2 8 0

Dose: 1 to 4 pills thrice a day after meals. Chief ingredients are Abhraka Bhasma, Makshika Bhasma, Trikatu, Triphala, Vidanga and Shilajatu. Diet: Milk and rice only. Alterative, tonic, hæmatinic. Specially suitable in phthisis, spermatorrhœa, diabetes, chyluria, Bright s disease, heart affections, scrofula, anæmia, dropsy. Removes general and sexual debility.

**Dashanga Gugula.**

Bhav.

Dose· 1 to 4 pills to be taken three times a day. Chief ingredients are Tr katu, Triphala, Chitraka and Gugulu .Alterative, tonic, stimulant. Specially suitable in obesity. Also useful in nervous and heumatic affections.

**Dadimivati.**

Nighant Part II.

Dose: 1 to 4 pills twice a day. Each pill contains 1/3 gr. Opium. Sole ingredi nts are Shunthi, opium, Jatiphala and Dadimatwak. Hypnotic, sedative, analgesic, hæmostatic. Useful in insomnia, excitement, delirium, neuralgic and abdominal pain, the pain of pleurisy, gastric ulcer, cancer, biliary and renal calculi, after pains, intestinal and pulmonary hæmorrhage, diabetes, diarrhœa, cholera, etc. It reduces the tendency to syncope and relieves angina pectora. Contra indicated in kidneys, chronic dyspepsia, coma, wi h contracted pupil, in nursing females and plethoric persons, in cerebral hyperæmia, in alcoholic intoxication, in advanced stages of bronchitis, pneumonia or whenever the respiration is seriously embarrassed.

**Pakshavadha Guggulu.**

Nighant Part II.

Dose: 1 to 4 pills, to be taken three times a day with Rasanadi Quath. Chief ingredients are

Guggulu, Triphala, Yavani, Sarshapa, Patha, Chitraka, Hingu, Indrayava, Jiraka, etc.

Alterative, tonic. Useful in paraplegia, hemiplegia, and other paralytic affections.

### Pathadi Gutika.

Ch. Chi. Ch. 8.

Dose: 1 to 4 pills to be taken three times a day. Sole ingredients are Patha, Yavani and Bilvapeshika. Astringent, gastric stimulant, tonic, antiseptic. Specially useful in diarrhœa of phthisis. Increases the flow of saliva, augments the gastric secretion and promotes appetite.

### Pradarari Loha.

Bhai.

Dose: 1 to 4 pills, to be taken twice a day with milk or water. Chief ingredients are Abhraka Bhasma, Loha Bhasma, Patha, Bilvapeshika, Kutajatwak, etc. Astringent, tonic, hæmatinic. Cures leucorrhœa, anæmia, Bright's disease, heart affections, scrofula, chronic diarrhœa, dysentery.

### Pleehari Vatika.

Bhai.

Dose: 1 to 3 pills at night after meals. Chief ingredients are aloes, Abhraka Bhasma, Kasisa and Lasuna. Tonic, hæmatinic. Useful in diseases of spleen and liver, dropsy, chlorosis, amenorrhœa, dysmenorrhœa. Contra-indicated in pregnancy and nursing stage.

### Balaguti.

Dose to a child, 1 to 3 months old, 1 pill once only; 3 to 6 months old, 2 pills once only; 6 to 12 months old, 3 pills twice a day; 12 to 24 months old, 4 pills twice a day; above that age 5 or more pills twice a day. These pills are non-poisonous, prepared from best vegetable drug. Gives strength to the infantile constitution and keeps the child healthy and robust. Cures diseases of children, as cold, diarrhœa, tympanitis, etc.

*Directions.*—Generally the pill is administered with mother's milk. It is given to stop diarrhœa, with Ativisha water; in tympanitis, with dill water; in constipation, with Haritaki water.

**Mandura Loha.**

**S. U. Ch. 44.**

Dose: 1 to 4 pills, to be taken twice a day after food. Chief ingredients are Trikatu, Chitraka, Vidanga, Makshika Bhasma and Mandoora Bhasma. Tonic, hæmatinic. Useful in giddiness, asthma, (between attacks), general debility, sexual debility, enlargement of spleen, fainting (between attacks), chyluria, scrofula, heart disease and wherever there is poverty of blood.

**Madhumeha Gutika.**

Dose: 1 to 4 pills twice a day after meals. Each pill contains 1/100 gr. arsenic and 1/4 gr. nux vomica. Specific for diabetes. Is useful in gastric neuralgia, vomiting of chronic alcoholism. Chief ingredients are Gudoochi Rasakriya, Vishatinduka (nux vomica), Iron and arsenic. It is valuable in chronic skin diseases, in malignant anæmia, chlorosis and scrofula.

**Madhumeha Gutika.**

Each pill contains 1/10 gr. opium. Dose; 1 to 4 pills, to be taken twice a day with water. Sole ingredients are Gudoochi Rasakriya, opium, Loha (iron) and Navasagar. Specific for diabetes. These two pills should be given alternately every week. For contra-indications see Dadimivati.

### Yogaraj Guggulu.

Sha. M. Ch. 7.

Dose: 1 to 4 pills, to be taken three times a day. Chief ingredients are Triphala, Guggulu, Vacha, Shunthi, Katuki, Pippali, Patha, Jiraka, Hingu, etc. Alterative, tonic. Useful in synovitis, paraplegia, sciatica, hemiplegia and other nervous affections.

### Rasna Guggulu.

Bhav.

Dose: 1 to 4 pills, to be taken three times a day. Sole ingredients are Rasna and Guggulu. Alterative, tonic. Useful in synovitis, sciatica, paraplegia, hemiplegia and other nervous affections.

### Lashunadi Vati.

Vaidya Jivan.

Dose: 1 to 4 pills, whenever desired. Chief ingredients are Trikatu, Jiraka, Ajmoda, Saindhava, Hingu and Lashuna. Stomachic, stimulant, carminative. Aids digestion. Is useful in loss of appetite, flatulence, tympanitis, etc.

### Lodhradi Gutika.

S. U. Ch. 40.

Dose: 1 to 4 pills, to be taken three times a day. Sole ingredients are Lodhra, Bida and Bilvapeshika. Alterative, astringent, tonic. Useful in chronic diarrhœa and dysentery and menorrhagia, etc.

### Loha Guggulu.

Bhav.

Dose: 1 to 4 pills, to be taken twice a day after food with milk. Chief ingredients are Loha Bhasma, Guggulu, Trikatu and Triphala. Tonic, hæmatinic. Useful in general debility, sexual debility, anæmia, chlorosis, heart affections, scrofula and debility of old age.

### Laxative Pills.

Dose: 1 to 4, to be taken at night. Contains the following ingredients. Res. Podoph. Ex. Hyocy., Ext. Tarax., Ex. Colc Co., Ex. Jalapæ., Res. Leptandrini. Laxative. Useful in liver complaints, indigestion, constipation, etc

### Vriddhibadhika Vati.

Dose: 1 to 4 pills, to be taken three times a day. Chief ingredients are Kuberaksha, Indrayava, Kindaru, Haritaki, etc. Alterative, tonic. Specially useful in orchitis. May be advantageously given between attacks for a long time.

### Shoathahar Loha.

Ch. Chi. Ch. 17.

Dose: 1 to 4 pills, to be taken three times a day after food. Sole ingredients are Trikatu, Loha Bhasma and Yavakshara. Tonic, hæmatinic, gastric stimulant, antacid. Valuable in dropsy due to anæmia; also useful in scrofula, Bright's disease, heart affections, phosphaturia, calculi, etc.

### Sanjivani Pills.

Sha. M. Ch. 7.

Dose: 1 to 4 pills, three times a day. Each pill contains 1/10 gr. aconite. Chief ingredients are Triphala, Shunthi, Pippali, Bhallataka, Aconite, Vacha, etc. Sedative and gastric stimulant. Useful in indigestion, chronic diarrhœa, cholera, etc.

### Saptasalivati.

Bhav.

Dose: 1 to 4 pills, to be taken after food. Each pill contains 1/7 gr. mercury. Chief ingredients are mercury, Khadirasara and Akarkarabha. Useful in infantile syphilis. One pill may be given to children in diseases attended with deficient biliary secretion. Is specially useful in allaying the childish ailment of vomiting after food. This pill when taken at night and followed by Samudrakavirechan Churna next morning proves beneficial in hepatic dyspepsia.

### Samshamani Pills.

Dose for children, 1 to 4 pills, dose for adults; 5 to 15 pills. To be taken three times a day. The sole ingredient is Gudoochi. Bitter tonic, antiperiodic. Most valuable in diseases of children, as diarrhœa, cold, general debility, etc. It is also given to children to improve health. Is also very useful in female complaints such as leucorrhœa. As bitter tonic, it is useful in atonic dyspepsia, feverishness and general debility.

*Directions.*—Given to children with mother's milk twice a day; in tympanitis with Dill water and in constipation with Haritaki water.

### Swayambhuva Guggulu.

Vag. U. Ch 28.

Dose: 1 to 4 pills, to be taken twice a day with Manjisthadi Quath. Chief ingredients are Guggulu, Triphala, Pippali, Twak and Ela. Alterative, tonic. Useful in abscesses, boils, ulcers, fistula, etc.

### Hinguadi Gutika.

Bang.

Dose: 1 to 4 pills taken two hours after meals. Chief ingredients are Hingu, Krishna Lavana, Patha, Yavakshara, Swarjika and Saindhava, etc. Antacid, carminative. Useful in heart-burn, hyperacidity, dyspepsia, enlargement of prostrate gland, rheumatism, uric acid diathesis and lumbago.

## Hingualiyadi Pills.

To be taken three times a day. Sole ingredients are Eliyaka and Hingu. Cathartic, tonic, carminative. Useful in amenorrhœa with constipation, flatulence, hepatic colic, tympanitis.

## Gonorrhœa Pills.

Dose: 1 to 4, to be taken three times a day. Chief ingredients are Chandana, Kankola and Guggula. Stimulant, carminative, diuretic, disinfectant. Specific for gonor hœa and gleet, bronchitis and laryngitis.

## TABLETS.

Tablets are a new feature in Ayurvaidic preparations. Medicines containing salts or sugars are easily made into tablets and such form has been appreciated by our constituents. We, however, supply the same preparation in both pill and tablet form. It should therefore be distinctly mentioned whether pill or tablet is required. The following rates are for tablets only. Those of pills vary with the items. Tablets are made of 1 to 20 grains weight according to the dose.

### Abhayadi Modak.

Sha. U. Ch.

Dose: 3 to 12 to be tak n as directed with warm water. Cathartic. Produces watery stools. Chief ingredients are Trivrit, Sugar, Dantimula, Pippali, Amalak, etc.

### Arkadi Tablets.

Dose: 2 to 6 tablets to be taken as directed. Each tablet contains 1/4 gr. opium. Sole ingredients are opium, Arkachurna and Potassium. Citrate. Alterative, sedative. Very valuable remedy in dysentery, chronic diarrhœa, cholera. Also useful in incipient colds and as an anodyne in gastric pain; cystitis, whooping cough, retention of urine, etc.

### Avipattikar Tablet.

Rasendra.

Dose: 2 to 8 tablets to be taken with cocoanut water. Chief ingredients are Trivrit, sugar, Lavanga, Trikatu, Triphala, etc. Purgative and carminative. Specially suitable in vomiting, hyperacidity, heart-burn, indigestion. Also beneficial in constipation, dropsy or Bright's disease; melancholia; rheumatic and paralytic affections. Contra-indicated when bowels are inflamed.

### Ashtang Lavana.

Ch. Chi. Ch. 12.

Dose: 1 to 4 tablets to be taken before or with food. Chief ingredients are Krishnalavana, Jiraka, Amlavetasa, Ela, Saindhava, Tintidika, etc. Stomachic, stimulant. Increases appetite, hence useful in anorexia, in gastric debility caused by alcoholism.

### Amalakyadi Vati.

Sha. M. Ch. 7.

Allow 1 to 4 tablets to dissolve in the mouth. 10 to 15 tablets may be taken during the whole day. Chief ingredients are Amalaka, Padma, Kustha, sugar, etc. Prescribed in Shastras for thirst.

### Ayushyavardhani.

(Amritsar Gutika) Rasa Ratna.

Dose: 1 to 4, to be taken twice after meals. Chief ingredients are Triphala, Gudoochi, Vriddhadaraka, Trikatu, Ela, etc. Alterative, aperient. Specially useful in piles, and in various diseases of chest, and in enlargement of abdominal viscera.

### Eladi Tablets.

Ch. Chi. Ch. 16.

Dose: 1 to 4, to be taken three times a day. Chief ingredients are Ela, Tamalpatra, Twak,

Yasthimadhu, Kharjura and Draksha. Nutritive, tonic, demulcent. Useful in general and sexual debility; it also acts beneficially on bronchial affections.

## Kanthya Tablets.

Dose: 1 to 3, to be sucked at a time. Sole ingredient is Potas. Chloras. An active remedy in stomatitis, tonsilitis, cough, chronic bronchitis, hoarseness of voice. A solution of 1 tablet in 1 oz. of water may be beneficially applied on unhealthy sores and ulcers, and may also be used to wash sinus: the powder may be applied on the spots of apthæ and spongy gums.

## Kasis Tablets.

V. U. Ch. 9.

A solution 1 tablet in 4 oz. of water is of 1 in 500 strength. If stronger solution is required, dissolve one tablet in two oz. water. The sole ingredient is Kasisa (Ferrus Sulphate). Astringent. Gives good results in erysipelas, and in injections in elephantiasis, prolapsus ani, etc. A solution of 1 tablet in 1 oz. water applied on the eyelids cures blepharitis. **For internal use.** 1 gr. tablet. Dose: 1 to 5 to be taken after meals. Tonic, hæmatinic, styptic, astringent, emmenagogue. Useful in bleeding of the nose, hæmoptysis, hæmatemesis, anæmia, amenorrhœa.

## Kasisadi Tikdi.

Sole ingredients are Kasisa, Surastraja, Kankola and sugar. A solution of 1 tablet in 1 oz. water should be applied to the inside of the throat in diphtheria.

## Krimighna Tablets.

Dose: 1 to 4, to be taken on an empty stomach followed after two, hours, by a brisk purgative as castor oil. The chief ingredient is Santonine. Anthelmintic. Used to destroy internal parasites round and thread worms. Each tablet contains 1 gr. of Santonine.

## Jantughna Tablets.

Each tablet contains 1/75 gr. (mercuric chloride) Rasakarpura. Chief ingredient is Rasakarpura. One tablet in 4 oz. water gives a solution of 1 in 1000. Disinfectant, antiseptic. Specific for all parasitic skin diseases. Solution (1 in 6000 to 12000) is useful for washing in pruritus vulvae, leucorrhœa, goitre, ulcers, ozœna; and solution (1 in 3000) is useful for washing syphilitic chancre. Solution (1 in 5000) is generally useful in eye diseases.

## Jantughna-Grahi Tablets.

Each tablet contains 1/10 gr. opium. One tablet in 11 oz. water gives a solution 1 in 500. Antiseptic and astringent. The solution is useful for washing in prolapsus ani, herpes, otalgia, pruritus ani, fissure of anus, chancre, sinus, leucorrhœa, stomatitis, etc.

## Tankanamla Tablets. (Boric Acid).

Chief ingredient is Tankanamla (Boric acid). For eye lotions, only distilled water should be used. An unirritating local antiseptic. Useful as a dressing for granulating and suppurating surfaces in general; as an eye wash, 4 to 8 grs. in 1 oz. water; as a lotion, douche or as a mouthwash 8 to 16 grs. to an oz. of water; as a paint for the throat 1 in 5 of glycerine; also useful as a dusting powder in pruritus vulvæ, etc.

## TABLETS.

### Tuttha Tikdi.

S. U. Ch. 12.

One tablet in 4 oz. water gives a solution 1 in 500. Chief ingredient is Tuttha (copper sulphate). Astringent, exharotic. 1 in 500 solution is a useful lotion for prurigo, lichen, granular conjunctivitis, etc. The powder of the tablet is useful as caustic for warts. For eye lotions, only distilled water should be used.

### Triphala Tablets.

Dose 2 to 8 tablets to be taken with milk. Chief ingredients are Haritaki, Bibhitaka and Amalaka. Alterative, astringent. Useful in hæmoptysis and other internal hæmorrhages. In conjunctivitis and other eye diseases, Triphala is extensively used internally as an alterative.

### Dashasar Tikdi. Rasratna.

Dose: 1 to 4 tablets, to be taken three times a day with water. Chief ingredients are Yastimadhu, Draksha, Amalaka, Ela, Chandana, Dadimbij and sugar. Demulcent, astringent, sedative. Useful in bleeding of the nose and other internal hæmorrhages; also in hematuria, gleet.

### Drakshadi Tikdi.

Yog.

Dose. 1 to 4 tablets to be taken three times a day with water. Chief ingredients are Draksha, Yastimadhu, Vanshalochana, Chandana, Kankola, Ela, Pippali, Valaka and sugar. Alterative; useful in vomiting, hematuria, epistaxis, gonorrhœa, gleet, bronchitis, laryngitis and general debility.

## Navsagar Tablets.

(Ammoni Chloridum.)

Dose: 1 to 4 tablets, to be taken three times a day with water. the chief ingredient is Navasagar. Hepatic, gastric and intestinal stimulant; diaphoretic and diuretic. Useful in acute and chronic congestion of the liver, neuralgia, lumbago, migraine, sciatica, gout, chronic rheumatism. In bronchitis, this should be kept in the mouth and be slowly sucked.

## Navayas Tikdi.

Nighant Part 2.

Dose: 1 to 4 to be taken three times a day after meals. Chief ingredients are Loha-Bhasma, Trikatu, Triphala, Lavanga, Jatiphala, and Ela. Hæmatinic, tonic, alterative. Specially suitable in phthisis: also in general and sexual debility, chyluria, scrofula, heart disease, anæmia, chlorosis, dropsy and all anæmic conditions.

## Pippali Modak.

Sha. M. Ch. 7.

Dose: 1 to 4, to be taken three times a day with milk. Chief ingredients are Pippali, sugar, milk and Chaturjat. Stimulant, tonic, nutritive. Useful in asthma, cough, dyspepsia and general debility.

## Punarnava Mandura.

Ch. Chi. Ch. 20.

Dose : 1 to 4 to be taken twice a day after food with milk. Chief ingredients are Mandura Bhasma, Punarnava, &c. Tonic, hæmatinic. Specially suitable for dropsy. Also in chlorosis, amenorrhœa, anæmia, scrofula, heart affections, general debility, sexual debility. In dropsy, these tablets should be taken with Punarnavadi Quath.

## TABLETS.

### Pranada Gutika.

Bhai.

Dose: 1 to 4, to be taken twice a day or once at night only with water. Chief ingredients are Haritaki, Shunthi, Maricha, Pippali, Pippalimoola and sugar. Laxative, alterative; useful in piles, dyspepsia, cough and constipation.

### No. 1315. Manduravatak.

Dose: 1 to 4, to be taken twice a day after food. Chief ingredients are Mandura, Trikatu, Triphala, Chitraka, Vidanga, &c. Tonic, hæmatinic Most useful in anæmia and incontinence of urine in children. Also useful in chlorosis, scrofula, heart affections, phthisis, general debility, sexual debility. This is specially given to anæmic children who eat earth.

### Marichadi Guti.

Dose: 1 to 4 tablets, to be kept in the mouth when suffering from cough. In other diseases, to be taken three times a day with water. Chief ingredients are Maricha, Pippali, Yavakshara, Dadim and sugar. Stimulant, antacid, diuretic, expectorant and uric acid solvent. Useful in dyspepsia, hyperacidity, heart-burn, cough, bronchitis, rheumatism, dysuria, calculi, etc.

### Mehantak (Gonorrhœa)

Chief ingredients are Sugar of Lead, Zinc Acetate, Rasanjan and opium. A solution of one tablet in 1 or 2 oz. of water is excellent for urethral and vaginal injection. Useful in sub-acute stages of gonorrhœa. Each tablet contains $\frac{1}{8}$ gr. opium.

### Yashthyadi Tikdi.

To be kept in the mouth, when necessary. The only ingredients are Navasagar and Yasthimadhu. Demulcent, expectorant. Useful in hoarseness, cough and bronchial catarrh.

**Lavangadi Vati**

Vaidya Jivan.

Allow it to dissolve in the mouth. Chief ingredients are Lavanga, Maricha, Bibhitaka and Khadirsar. Demulcent. This is a popular medicine for cough.

**Vyoshadi Guti.**

Sha. M. Ch. 7'

To be kept in the mouth and slowly dissolved. Chief ingredients are Trikatu, Amlavetasa, Chitraka, Jiraka. Stimulant. Useful in cold, cough, bronchitis, indigestion, etc.

**Shiva-Kshar-pachan Vati.**

Dose: 2 to 6, to be taken with water twice a day, Chief ingredients are Shiva, Swarjika-kshara and Hinguastak Churna. Mild purgative and gastric stimulant. Useful in colic, indigestion, dyspepsia, heartburn, vomiting, acidity, tympanitis, constipation, headache, cholera, etc.

**Shital Powder.**

To be dissolved in water 1½ times the weight of the powder and the water will begin to cool slowly, finally going to —12°c (cooler than ice). If dissolved in equal parts of water, it cools upto—24°c. Chief ingredients are Navasagar and Suryakshara. Useful as a cooling lotion in prurigo, bubo, fevers, abscess, and all burning or inflammatory affections.

**Shunthyadi Tikdi.**

Dose : 1 to 4, to be taken three times a day. Chief ingredients are Shunthi and Swarjika. Gastric stimulant, antacid. Useful in hyperacidity, hiccough, dyspepsia, heart-burn, nausea, vomiting, rheumatism, &c.

## TABLETS.

### Sitopaladi Tablets.

Sha. M. Ch. VI.

Dose: 2 to 8, to be taken as desired. Chief ingredients are Ela, Pippali, Vanshlochan and sugar. Expectorant, stimulant. Useful in cough, bronchitis, phthisis and other chest affections and burning of the feet.

### Surastraja Tablets.

One tablet in 4 oz. of water gives a solution of 1 in 500, which will be ordinarily useful. The chief ingredient is Surastraja (alum). Recommended for local wash in pruritus vulvæ, fissure of the anus, tonsilitis, epistaxis, ozœna, etc.

### Sooranvatak.

Sha. M. Ch. VII.

Dose: 1 to 4, to be taken three times a day with water. Chief ingredients are Surana, Chitraka, Shunthi, Maricha. Alterative, stimulant. Specially suitable for piles. Being helpful in digestion, is useful in dyspepsia, chronic diarrhœa, asthma, cough, hiccough, enlargement of spleen, sexual debility.

### Sooranvatak (Brihat).

Sha. M. Ch. 7.

Dose : 1 to 4, to be taken three times a day with whey. Chief ingredients are Surana, Chitraka, Vriddhadaraka, Musali, Bhallataka, &c. Alterative, stomachic; specially suitable in piles. Promotes appetite, helps digestion. Is also useful in chronic diarrhœa, dyspepsia, asthma, cough, enlargement of the spleen, hiccough, sexual debility, &c.

### Saindhavadi Tablets.

Ch. Chi. Ch. 16.

Dose : 1 to 4 tablets, to be taken before or with

food. Chief ingredients are Saindhava, Krishnalavana, Dadima, Jiraka, Dhanyak, sugar, Phalamla. Carminative, gastric stimulant, Useful in loss of appetite, indigestion, anorexia of phthisis, alcoholism.

## Sodawater Tablets.

To be taken when required with water. Chief ingredient are Soda Bicarb, Citric Acid and Tartaric Acid. Useful as sodawater in vomiting, thirst, gout, dyspepsia, etc.

## Headache Cure Tablets.

Two tablets followed by hot tea or coffee will immediately relieve the pain. Chief ingredients are Caffeina Citras and Phenacitin. Analgesic. Very efficacious in headache, neuralgia and migrane.

---

## AVALEHAS (Confections.)

The following Avalehas are prepared according to Shastras. In Chyavanprash, especially, we have fixed the proportion of Amalakas, in weight as against numbers, and a proportionate part of sugar is mixed. In all other respects, the Shastriya formula is strictly adhered to.

### Agastyaharitakee Avaleha

Sha. M. Ch. 8.

Dose: one half to one tola, to be given every morning followed by milk. Chief ingredients are Haritaki, Yava, Dashamoola, Chitraka, Pippali. Alterative and nutritive. Useful in cough, hiccough, asthma, piles, phthisis and general debility. Diet: milk and rice.

### Abhayamalaki (Brahmya-Rasayan).

Ch. Chi. Ch. I. V. 54.

Dose: ¼ to 1 tola, to be taken in the morning with milk. Chief ingredients are Haritaki, Amalaka, Brahmi, Shankhpushpi, Vidanga, Chandana, Agaru, Vacha, Dashamoola, etc. Alterative, tonic. Specially suitable for debility of old age and general debility accompanied with mental weakness or weak memory.

### Amritbhallatak.

Bhav. M. Kushta.

Dose: ⅛ to ½ tola, to be taken twice a day with milk. Chief ingredients are Bhallatak, Gudoochi. Alterative, stimulant, nervine tonic. Recommended in Ayurvedic books for leprosy, scrofula and venereal diseases and sexual debility: Avoid Capsicum and pungent spices; also sun heat and fire.

### Kantakarya Avaleha.

Sha. M. Ch. VIII.

Dose: ½ to 2 tolas, to be taken when necessary,

followed by milk. Chief ingredients are Kantakari, Chitraka, Shringi, Trikatu, Rasna, etc. Expectorant, diuretic and aperient. Useful in cough, bronchitis, asthma and other chest diseases. Is also useful as diuretic in disuria and dropsy.

**Kutajawaleha.**

Sha. M. Ch. 8.

Dose: ¼ to 1 tola, to be taken three times a day with whey. Chief ingredients are Kutajatwak, Trikatu, Trifala, Bhallataka, etc. Astringent and antiperiodic. Very useful in dysentery, chronic diarrhœa, hematemesis, melæna, vomiting, bleeding piles, chronic dyspepsia.

**Gokshuradyavaleha.**

Sha. M. Ch. 8.

Dose: ½ to 1 tola, to be taken with milk three times a day. Chief ingredients are Gokshuraka, Trikatu, Trapusha, Kasha, etc. Demulcent, diuretic, tonic. Relieves painful micturition and increases the flow of urine. Useful in dysuria, cystitis, calculi, incontinence of urine and other urinary and calculus affections. It is also useful in gonorrhœa and gleet, nocturnal emissions and sexual debility.

**Chyavanprash (Jivan).**

Sha. M. Ch. 8.

Dose: ½ to 2 tolas, to be taken every morning with milk. Chief ingredients are Amalaka, Dashamoola, Pippali, Vanshlochan, &c. Nutritive, tonic; strengthens the constitution. Very useful as a nutritive in phthisis, general debility, cough, hoarseness of voice, debility of old age. In short, this very popular Avaleha improves all conditions of debility.

**Dhatryavaleha.**

Ch. Chi. Ch. 20.

Dose: ¼ to 1 tola, to be taken with milk or whey twice or thrice a day. Chief ingredients are

Amalaka, Yastimadhu, Vanshlochan, Pippali, &c. Alterative, stimulant, demulcent. Specially suitable in cough, bronchitis and other chest affections.

**Pippalyadileha.**

Va. Chi. Ch. 16.

Dose : ½ to 1 tola, to be taken with milk twice or thrice a day. Chief ingredients are Pippali, Draksha, Yastimadhu, Amalaka. Demulcent, expectorant and aperient ; alterative and stimulant. Useful in chest affections as bronchitis, phthisis and chronic cough and dyspepsia, enlargement of the spleen, constipation, &c.

**Brihan-Narikelkhand.**

Bhai R. Amlapittadhikar.

Dose : ½ to 1 tola, to be taken twice a day. Chief ingredients are Narikela, Shunthi, and sugar. Alterative. Specially suitable in hyperacidity, vomiting, intestinal colic, intestinal hæmorrhage, &c.

**Vasaleha.**

Bhav. Rajyakshma.

Dose: ½ to 1 tola, to be taken with milk when required. Chief ingredients are Vasa and Pippali. Expectorant, antispasmodic, alterative. Most valuable medicine in bronchitis. It is used with advantage in phthisis, asthma and other chest affections attended with cough and hectic fever. Stops blood in hæmoptysis and other internal hæmorrhages

**Vasavaleha.** Gad.

Dose: ½ to 1 tola, to be taken when required with milk. Chief ingredients are Vasa, Haritaki, Vanshalochan and Pippali. Expectorant, antispasmodic, alterative, astringent. Uses : same as above with this difference that as this contains Haritaki, it is more effective in chest affections attended with hæmorrhages.

### Vidangsaravaleha.

Vag. U. Ch. 28.

**Dose: ½ to 2 tolas, to be taken twice a day with Manjisthadi Quath. Chief ingredients are Vidanga, Pippali and Triphala. Anthelmintic. Useful in worms, fistula et ano, sinus, urinary diseases, ulcers, leprosy and other skin affections.**

### Vidangadyavaleha.

Gad. Nigraha

**Dose; ⅛ to ¼ tola, twice a day after food. Chief ingredients are Vidanga, Triphala, Yastimadhu, Katuki and Loha Bhasma. Alterative, tonic. Useful in thread worms, anæmia, jaundice, dropsy and general debility.**

### Shrirag.

**Dose: ¼ to 1 tola, to be taken three or four times a day with whey. The chief ingredient is Bilva. Astringent. Most valuable in chronic diarrhœa, diarrhœa, dysentery, infantile dysentery and sprue.**

### Salsaradyavaleha.

S. Chi. Ch. 12.

**Dose: 10 to 40 grains, to be taken three times a day after food. Chief ingredients are Tamra Bhasma, Loha Bhasma, decoction of Salsaradigana, Amalaka and Lodhra. Alterative tonic. Specially suitable in diabetes melitus.**

### Swadishta Chatan.

**Dose: ⅛ to ½ tola, when desired, before or with meals. Chief ingredients are Trikatu, Jirak, Sauvarchala and Lemon Juice. Stomachic, stimulant. Useful in loss of appetite, indigestion, tympanitis, dyspepsia, &c.**

## AVALEHAS (Confections.)

### Vyaghri Haritaki Avaleha.

**Ni. R. Part 2.**

**Dose: ½ to 2 tolas. Chief ingredients are Haritaki, Kantakarika. Expectorant, astringent. Extensively used in hiccough, cough, brcnchitis, asthma, and other chest affections.**

---

## GHRITAS.

In ancient medical books of Charaka and Susruta, are found more preparations of Ghritas than those of powders and pills. Thus it appears that physicians of those days were using Ghrita preparations in most cases. But what suited our Ancients, does not suit our refined moderns. We therefore, select only some limited preparations of Ghrita.

Ghritas do not require any Anupan. Wherever milk is prescribed, it is to be taken after the regular dose of the medicine.

The dose of the Ghritas should be determined according to the digesting power of the patient. Our Ghrita preparations are made from fresh and best Ghrita and are adapted for internal use.

Ghritas for application purposes are made according to Shastriya formulæ, and these are for the most part to be filled up in ulcers. These Ghritas are meant to serve the purpose of destroying and preventing putrefaction, and to hasten the healing up of the ulcer. But the Ghrita itself is liable to decomposition, and hence there is some danger of mixing those medicines having the property of preventing putrefaction with a substance liable to decomposition.

We have therefore thought it desirable to mix the ingredients with simple ointment in lieu of Ghrita, and this preparation therefore possesses more healing properties than the Ghritas themselves. We stock both kinds of preparations and supply them to order.

### Asoka Ghrit.

Bhai.

Dose: ½ to 1 tola, to be taken twice a day with rice water. Alterative. Useful in Leucorrhœa, menorrhagia and other female complaints.

### Kalyanaka Ghrit.

Ch. Chi. Ch. 14.

Dose: ½ to 2 tolas, to be taken twice a day with milk. Chief ingredients are Triphala, Deodar, Rasna, Punarnava, Darvi, Sariva, Vidanga, Kustha, etc. Alterative. Useful in Aphonia, mania, epilepsy, etc.

### Kasisadi Ghrit.

Sha. M. Ch. 9.

Chief ingredients are Kasisa, Haritala, Manashila, Tuttha, Sarshapa, Lodhra, Chakramarda, Karanjabij, &c. This Ghrit is useful as an application in ulcers, soft chancre, fissure of anus, fistula, piles, etc. This should be applied on the affected part, or a round cotton wick soaked in this Ghrita should be inserted in the punctured part. For Kasisadi Ointment see "Ointments."

### Chavyadi Ghrita.

Cha. Chi. Ch. 10.

Dose: ¼ to 1 tola, to be taken twice a day. Chie ingredients are Chavya, Trikatu, Pippalimoola, Yavani, Chitraka, Dadimatwak. Alterative, stomachic, stimulant, carminative; mild aperient. Specially suitable in cases of prolapsus ani, diarrhœa; gives strength to the intestines.

### Changeri Ghrit.

Sha. M. Ch. 9.

Dose: ¼ to 1 tola, to be taken twice a day with whey. Chief ingredients are Changeri, Yavani, Pippali, Pippalimoola, Chitraka, Gokshuraka, Bilvapeshika. Alterative, intestinal tonic, stimulant. Stops diarrhœa, gives strength to the intestines, and is specially suitable in prolapsus ani.

## Jatyadi Ghrita.

Sha. M. Ch. 9.

Chief ingredients are Jatipatra, Nimbapatra, Tuttha, &c. Styptic and local stimulant; escharotic. Very valuable for local use in all kinds of ulcers, sluggish sores, chancres, bleeding surfaces, fistula, etc.

## Tilwak Ghrit.

Su. U. Ch. 17.

Dose: ¼ to 1 tola, to be taken twice a day with milk. The chief ingredient is Lodhra. Alterative, tonic, as ringent. Specially suitable in night-blindness and other ye diseases. This is particularly beneficial when bowels are loose.

## Triphala Ghrita.

Sha. M. Ch. 9.

Dose: ¼ to 1 tola, to be taken in the morning with milk. Chief ingredients are Triphala, Vasa, Bhringaraja, &c. Alterative to ic. Useful in conjunctivitis and other eye diseases.

## Phala Ghrita.

Sha. M. Ch. 9.

Dose: ¼ to 1 tola, to be taken twice a day with milk. Chief ingredients are Triphala, Kustha, Katuki, Vacha, Sariva, Rasna, Vanshlochana, &c. Useful in sexual debility and sterility in women.

## Brahmi Ghrit.

Cha. Chi. Ch. 5.

Dose: ¼ to 1 tola, to be taken twice a day with milk on a empty stomach. The chief ingredient is Brahmi. Alterative, diuretic, stimulant. Most valuable in mania and epilepsy. It is also useful in aphonia and hoarseness of voice.

### Mahatikta Ghrita.

Sha. M. Ch. 9.

Dose : ½ to 2 tolas, to be taken twice a day. Chief ingredients are Saptaparna, Katuki, Patha, Parpat, Moorva, Vasa, Sariva and other bitter tonics. Bitter tonic, alterative. Recommended for leprosy.

### Lashoonadi Ghrita.

Cha. Chi. Ch. 14.

Dose : ¼ to 1 tola, to be taken three times a day. Chief ingredients ar Lashuna, Trikatu, Haritaki, and Hingu. Stimulant, carminative. Helps digestion, and promotes the flow of menses. Specially suitable in mania and amenorrhœa, hysteria, &c.

### Saraswat Ghrita.

Bang.

Dose : ¼ to 1 tola, to be taken twice a day. Chief ingredients are Shigrutwak, Vacha, Lodhra, Patha, Saindhava, etc. Bitter tonic, stimulant; adapted for aphonia and hoarseness of voice.

### Siddharthaka Ghrita.

Y. R. Unmad.

Dose : ¼ to 1 tola, to be taken twice a day. Chief ingredients are Sidhharthaka, Vacha, Hingu, Trikatu, Darvi, Deodara, etc. Stimulant, alterative. Specially suitable in pilepsy and mania.

### Hinguadi Ghrita.

Cha. Chi. Ch. 14.

Dose : ¼ to 1 tola, to be taken twice a day. Chief ingredients are Hingu, Brahmi, Sinduvara and Hingupatri. Alterative, stimulant and carminative. Specially suitable in mania, epilepsy, hysteria and other nervous complaints.

## OINTMENTS.

As mentioned in the general instructions at the head of Ghritas, we have prepared ointments of Kasisadi and Jatyadi Ghritas; and we are sure that this change will bc appreciated by the physician. Moreover, the ointment is more adapted in cases of prurigo, ringworm and eczema and below will be found some useful preparations of ointments.

### Ahiphenadi Ointment.

To be applied on the painful part. Chief ingredients are opium and galls. Anodyne. Useful for external application in hemorrhoids, fistula et ano and other painful inflammations.

### Kasisadi Ointment.

Same as Kasisadi Ghrit. This is useful as an application in ulcers, soft chancre, fissure of anus, fistula, piles, etc. This ointment has been prepared by using simple ointment instead of Ghrita, owing to the latter's tendency to putrify. Otherwise the Shastriya formula has been followed to the letter.

### Gandhaka Ointment.

The chief ingredient is Gandhaka (Sulphur). Useful in scabies. The affected part should be thoroughly cleansed with carbolic soap and warm water, after which the ointment to be rubbed in.

### Jasata Ointment.

Chief ingredients are Jasatapushpa (Zinc oxide) and simple ointment. Mild astringent. Useful in blepharitis, eczema and ulceration.

### Jatyadi Ointment.

Sha. M. Ch. 9.

This ointment is prepared according to the formula for Jatyadi Ghrita with the only difference that simple ointment has been used instead of Ghrita. Styptic and local stimulant. Very valuable for local use in all kinds of ulcers, such as carbuncle, soft chancre, fistula, It stops suppuration; heals the part very quickly.

### Turushkadi Ointment.

Chief ingredients are Jasatapushpa, Boric acid and Turushka. Astringent, antiseptic. The ointment is a good remedy for eczema, chancre. To be applied in eczema after removing the crusts by poultice.

### Dadrughna (Ringworm) Ointment.

Chief ingredient is Rasakarpura (Mercuric Chloride). Disinfectant, escharotic, alterative. Useful in ringworm and eczema, psoriasis and other chronic and parasitic skin diseases. The affected part should be first thoroughly washed with soap, hot water, and then the ointment should be vigorously rubbed over.

### Paradadi Ointment.

The chief ingredient is Parada (mercury). Useful in parasitic skin diseases, such as ringworm of the scalp, scabies, chancre, &c.

### Snigdha Ointment.

Chief ingredients are oil of Theobroma and white wax. Deodorant, antiseptic. Useful for local use, as skin massage to keep it smooth in chicken-pox, prurigo, etc.

## TAILA (Medicated Oils).

In old medical books, Tailas are prescribed not only for application, but for internal use also. We are not sure whether the modern physicians prescribe Tailas for internal use. We have, therefore, not given below the proportion of dose to be taken internally. But if any physician thinks it desirable to give the dose internally, he may fix it himself.

When the oil is to be dropped into the ear, it should be warm enough.

---

### Apamarga Taila.

Bangsen.

Chief ingredients are Apamarga-bija, Trikatu, Yavakshara, Hingu and Vidanga. Sternutatory. Useful in hemicrania, headache, &c.

### Avalgujadi Taila.

Chief ingredients are Bakuchi, Kustha, Valaka, etc. The oil is to be applied on the part affected thrice a day. Most beneficial in Pityriasis and other skin diseases, such as ringworm of the scalp, psoriasis, etc.

### Adityapaka Taila.

Bhav. Kustha.

Chief ingredients are Manjistha, Triphala, Laksha, Gandhaka, etc. A certain cure for scabies. The ointment should be rubbed vigorously on the affected part after thoroughly washing it with carbolic soap and hot water.

### Irimedadi Taila.

Sha. M. Ch. 9.

Chief ingredients are Irimeda, Karpura, Lavanga, Kankola, Ela, Lodhra, Agaru, etc. Mild rubefacient, astringent, anesthetic, and antiseptic.

## TAILA (Medicated Oils).

In neuralgia, this oil should be vigorously rubbed on the affected part; in tooth-ache, the oil should be applied by soaking it in cotton and applying it to the affected part; in apthæ and other mouth diseases, it should be used as a gargle.

### Kanaka Taila.

Bang. Kshudra.

To be applied on the affected part. Chief ingredients are Yastimadhu, Manjistha, Priyangu, Chandana and Kanaka. Disinfectant, emollient and anodyne. Useful in acne and other skin diseases.

### Kasisadi Taila.

Sha. M. Ch. IX.

For external application only. Chief ingredients are Kasisa, Kustha, Saindhava, Vidanga, Chitraka, Haritala, Arkakshira, Snuhi-Kshira, etc. Very useful in pruritus ani, piles, ozœna, &c.

### Gunja Taila.

Bhav. Gandmala.

Useful as an application in scrofula. Chief ingredients are Gunjamoola and Gunja.

### Chakramarda Taila.

Bhav. Gandmal.

Recommended in Shastras for external application in scrofula. Chief ingredients are Chakramarda and Bhringaraj. Useful in eczema, pityrisis, ringworm, psoriasis and other skin diseases.

### Chandanadi Taila.

Yoga Ratna. Urahkshat.

Chief ingredients are Chandana, Nakha, Kustha, Agaru, Lavanga, Kumkuma, Laksha rasa, Manjistha, Pootikeshara, etc. Useful as an application in hemicrania, burning of the feet, headache, neuralgia, bleeding of the nose. In bleeding of nose, the oil should be applied on the head as well as in the nose. This oil has also been internally prescribed in cases of hæmoptysis.

No. 1729. **Chitrakadi Taila.**

Su. Chi. Ch. VIII.

Chief ingredients are Chitraka, Arkamoola, Trivrit, Patha, Udumbara, Vacha, Swarjika, Jyotishmati. Useful as an application in fistula, sinus and other deep ulcers. A cotton wick soaked in this oil should be put in the ulcers.

**Jatyadi Taila.**

Sha. M. Ch. IX.

Chief ingredients are Jatipallav, Nimbapatra, Patola Patra, Kustha, Yastimadhu, Manjistha, Lodhra, Tuttha, etc. Useful for local application in pruritus ani, fistula, sinus and deep ulcers.

**Narayan Taila.**

Sha. M. Ch. IX.

Chief ingredients are Shatavari, Ashwagandha, Bilvamoola, Patala, Gokshuraka, Syonaka, Agnimanth, etc. Highly recommended in Ayurvedic Shastras as a local massage in hemiplegia, lumbago, impotence, fever, phthisis, headache, paraplegia.

**Parvativilas (Dhustur) Taila.**

Bhaishajya : Shiroroga.

Chief ingredient is Dhustura. Anodyne. Useful for local application in sciatica, otalgia, inflammation of the ear, herpes, neuralgia and other painful affections.

**Manjisthadi Taila.**

Bangsen, Kshudraroga.

To be applied locally. Chief ingredients are Manjistha, Yastimadhu, Lodhra, Padmaka, Chandana, Laksha. Prescribed in Shastras for acne and skin affections.

## TAILA (Medicated Oils).

### Magadhyadi Taila.

Su. Chi. Ch. VIII.

Chief ingredients are Pippali, Lodhra, Kustha, Manjistha, Sariva, Padmaka, Vacha. Useful as an application in ulcers of fistula, sinus, scrofula, etc.

### Rasakarpuradi Taila.

Chief ingredient is Rasakarpur. A useful application to syphilitic sores, prurigo, eczema, goitre, orchitis, etc.

### Lashunadi Sneha (Taila).

Su. U. Ch. XXI.

Chief ingredients are Lashuna, Shigrutwak, Moolakawater, Kadaliwater. Local irritant and stimulant. A useful application in earache.

### Lakshadi Taila.

Sha. M. Ch. IX.

Chief ingredients are Laksha, Aswagandha, Deodar, Katuki, Chandana, Moorva. A very useful remedy as a massage in fevers, cough, asthma, cold, epilepsy, mania and phthisis.

### Vidang Taila.

Bangsen. Shiroroga.

Chief ingredients are Vidanga, Dantimoola and Swarjika. To be applied to the forehead or dropped into the nose. Sternutatory. Relieves severe headache. Useful in hemicrania.

### Vishagarbha Taila.

Ni. Ratna. Part II. Vatroga.

Chief ingredients are Nirgundi water, Bhringraj water, Dhustura and aconite. Anodyne. Sedative. Relieves pain of any kind. Useful in hemicrania, earache, inflammation of the ear, paraplagia, sciatica, neuralgia, lumbago, gout, bubo, rheumatism, colic, and other painful inflammatory affections.

### Shwetadi Taila.

Su. Chi. Ch. XXII.

Chief ingredients are Shweta, Dantimoola, Vidanga. Useful as a gargle in diphtheria.

### Haridradi Taila.

Bangsen, Kshudraroga.

Chief ingredients are Haridra, Agaru, Darvi, Manjistha, Padma, etc. A useful application in acne.

### Hinguadi Taila.

Su. U. Ch. XXIII.

Chief ingredients are Hingu, Trikatu, Indrayava, Laksha, Punarnava, Karanja, Vacha, Shigru. Three or four drops in the nose will bring relief in cases of ozœna.

## RASAS (Mercurial Preparations).

**General Directions :**—We have classed in Rasa all the preparations containing mercury in any form. And as most of these preparations contain various kinds of poisons, they are made into pills and tablets to facililate the proportion of dose.

Very much care is taken in the mixing of these poisons with other drugs. The dose marked for each such preparation is perfectly harmless and can be taken with the utmost safety.

We have mentioned the exact proportion of poisons occurring in each pill or tablet, and as these are of a uniform weight, the prescriber is able to give the desired dose to his patient.

Rasas are generally taken with quath, milk or water. These **Anupans** help in swallowing the medicines with ease

It is a general and an erroneous belief that very strict regimen must be observed during the continuance of the Rasa treatment; and that serious consequences follow any failure to observe the directions strictly. But our Rasas are quite harmless. Of course, wherever, any special directions have been given they have to be followed very strictly. Care must also be taken to observe all the diet instructions given by the physicians or mentioned in this book. General restrictions to avoid over eating so as to cause indigestion and pungent things in diet, are to be observed. They have no connection with either the disease or dietitic instructions.

For the most part, pills or tablets of these Rasas are made in smaller weights of 1 or 2 grains; thus enabling the physician to prescribe the smallest dose.

### Agnikumara Rasa.

Bhav. Jathar.

Dose, 1 to 2 pills as directed. Each pill contains 1/6 gr. aconite. Chief ingredients are Kajjali,

Trikatu, Swarjika, Shankh Bhasma and aconite. Sedative, stomachic, antacid. Useful in cholera colic, diarrhœa, indigestion, tympanitis.

For contra indications : see Sanjivani Gutika.

### Agnitundi Vati.

Sha. M. Ch. XII.

Dose, 1 to 4 pills with milk or water, after meals. Each pill contains 1/2 gr. nux vomica and 1/36 gr. aconite. Chief ingredients are Kajjali, Trikatu, Chitraka, two Ksharas, etc. Bitter, stomachic, tonic and stimulant. Stimulates the bowels and increases nervous energy ; is, therefore, useful in dyspepsia, indigestion, colic, heart weakness, neuralgia, lumbago, anæmia, sexual debility, diabetes, etc., and as a general tonic in all conditions of debility.

### Agni Rasa.

Rasa Ratna. Ch. XIII.

Dose 20 to 60 grs. to be taken with honey three times a day followed by milk. Chief ingredients are Kajjali, Haritaki, Pippali, Bibhitakatwak, Yastimadhu, Vasa. Alterative, tonic, demulcent, expectorant and anti-spasmodic. A specific for bronchitis and useful in the treatment of catarrhs, hoarseness of voice, asthma, pneumonia, croup, phthisis, and other chest diseases.

### Agnisoot Rasa.

Vai. Sa. Sam.

Dose 2 to 8 pills three times a day with rice, water or whey. Chief ingredients are Kajjali, Shankha Bhasma, Kapardi Bhasma, and Maricha. Gastric stimulant, antiseptic. Useful in dyspepsia diarrhœa, dysentery, colic, indigestion.

### Abhrakadi Vati.

Nighant Part II.

Dose, 1 to 4 pills, three times a day with milk. Each pill contains 1/16 gr. aconite and 1/16 gr.

opium. Chief ingredients are Kajjali, Loha Bhasma, Abhrak Bhasma and Trikatu.

Alterative, sedative, tonic. Specially useful in phthisis.

For contra-indications, see Sanjivani Gutika and Dadimi Vati.

### Amar Sundari Vati.

Nighant R. Part II.

Dose, 1 to 4 pills to be taken three times a day with water. Chief ingredients are Kajjali, Loha Bhasma, Trikatu, Triphala, Chaturjata, Musta, Akar-Karabha, sugar, etc. Alterative, stomachic, stimulant; tonic, anodyne, diaphoretic and diuretic. Useful in hysteria, epilepsy and other nervous diseases.

### Arshakuthara Rasa.

Rasasar Samgraha.

Dose, 1 to 4 pills three times a day with whey. Chief ingredients are Kajjali, Tamra Bhasma, Loha Bhasma, Trikatu, Surana, Yavakshara, etc. Alterative, tonic, laxative. Specially prescribed in piles. Gives tone to the body and keeps the bowels free.

### Ashwakanchuki Rasa.

Rasa Prakash Sudhaker.

Dose, 1 to 4 pills, when necessary, with water or molasses. Each pill contains 1-20 gr. croton seeds and 1/10 gr. aconite. Chief ingredients are Kajjali, Trikatu, Trifala, aconite and croton seeds. Purgative, calmative and diaphoretic; produces watery stools. Largely used in fevers and all other conditions, where a safe purgative and a diaphoretic is needed.

For contra-indications, see Sanjivani Guti.

**Anand Bhairav Rasa.**

Sha. M. Ch. XII.

Dose, 1 to 2 pills, to be taken twice a day with whey and Shakrayava Churna. Each pill contains 1/7 gr. aconite. Chief ingredients are Rasasindura, aconite, Tankana, Maricha and Pippali. Anodyne, diaphoretic, diuretic. Useful in chronic diarrhœa, nervous debility of old age, angina pectoris (between attacks).

For contra-indications, see Sanjivani Guti.

**Aarogya Vardhani.**

Rasa Ratna. Ch. XX.

Dose, 1 to 4 pills to be taken three times a day, with milk. Chief ingredients are Kajjali, Loha Bhasma, Abhrak Bhasma, Tamra Bhasma, Trifala, Shilajatu, Guggulu, Chitrak and Katuki. Alterative, aperient, tonic. Extensively used in jaundice, congestion of the liver, hepatitis, anæmia, enlargement of the spleen, dyspepsia and dropsy. In dropsy, this pill with only milk diet, effects certain cure in a short period.

**Ichhabhedi Rasa.**

Sha. M. Ch. XII.

Dose, 1 to 4 pills, whenever desired. Each pill contains 1/5 gr. croton seeds. Chief ingredients are Rasasindura, Tankana, Shunthi, Pippali, Hemakshirimool and croton seeds. Powerful hydragogue cathartic. Useful in obstinate constipation, dropsy, paralysis, and all other conditions where a powerful cathartic is needed.

Contra-indicated in feeble patients; also in cases of organic obstruction, or inflammatory condition of the stomach and intestines.

**Ekangaveera Rasa.**

Nighant Part II.

Dose, 1 to 4 pills, to be taken twice a day with Rasnadi Quath. Chief ingredients are Kajjali,

Banga Bhasma, Loha Bhasma, Naga Bhasma, Tamra Bhasma, Abhraka Bhasma, Vishatinduka, etc. Each pill contains 1/6 gr. nux vomica. Tonic, alterative. Useful in hemiplegia, paraplegia, paralysis, synovitis of the knee joints, sciatica.

### Kanak Sundara Rasa.

Nighant Part II.

Dose, 1 to 3 pills, three times a day with sugar. Each pill contains 1/3 gr. Datura seeds. Chief ingredients are Kajjali and Datura seeds. Diuretic, antispasmodic and anodyne. A very useful remedy in neuralgia, colic, asthma, dysmenorrhœa, retention of urine, cancer, whooping cough, acute sore throat and other painful affections.

### Kalkoota Rasa.

Vaid Sar. Samgraha.

Dose, 1 to 3 pills, 3 times a day with betel leaves. Each pill contains 1/7 gr. aconite. Chief ingredients are aconite, Kajjali, Tamra Bhasma, Manashila, Haratal, Chitrak and Triphala. To be taken in cases of fevers with mental derangement. In high fevers, it reduces temperature, and when given in paroxysm, acts as an antiperiodic.

For contra indications, see Sanjivani Guti

### Kravyada Rasa.

Yoga Ratna. Gulma.

Dose, 5 to 20 grs. to be taken when necessary with water. Chief ingredients are Takra, Jambira Rasa, Trifala, Chitraka, Ela, Shunthi, Saindhava, etc. Stomachic, stimulant, carminative. Useful in indigestion, tympanitis, diarrhœa, cholera, scurvy, typhoid fever, etc.

### Krimi Kuthara Rasa.

Nighant Part II.

Dose, 1 to 3 tablets, every one or two hours as desired. Each tablet contains 1/15 gr. aconite and 1 gr. camphor. Chief ingredients are Karpura, Rasa Sindura, Yavani, Kutaja, Trayanti, Vidanga, etc. Sedative, anti-spasmodic, diaphoretic and carminative. Specific for Cholera. Also useful in indigestion, tympanitis, cough, fever, dysmenorrhœa, angina pectoris, whooping cough, hysteria, etc.

### Krimimudgara Rasa.

Nighant Part II.

To be taken on an empty stomach 1 to 4 pills at a time and followed by a purgative, such as castor oil. Chief ingredients are Kajjali, Vidanga, Ajmoda, Mahanimba Bija and Palash Bija, &c. Useful in worms.

### Gandmalakandan Rasa.

Yoga Ratna.

Dose, 3 to 12 pills, twice a day with Manjisthadi quath. Chief ingredients are Kajjali, Tamra Bhasma, Loha Bhasma, Kanchanar bark and Guggulu. Alterative, tonic, hæmatinic. Specially efficacious in scrofulous affections ; improves general health, and restores the blood to its normal condition.

### Gandhaka Rasayan.

Yoga Ratna.

Dose, 5 to 20 grs. to be taken with sugar every night followed by milk. Chief ingredient is Gandhaka. Mild, laxative, alterative. Purifies blood. Useful in scabies, piles, prolapsus ani, chronic gout, chronic rheumatism, pruritus ani, prurigo.

Diet Restrictions :—Salt, acid, oil and mustard should be avoided.

### Garbhapal Rasa.

Vaid Sar Samgraha.

Dose, 1 to 4 pills, to be taken twice a day with milk or water. Chief ingredients are Naga Bhasma,

Bang Bhasma, Loha Bhasma, Rasasindur, ginger and other stomachics. Tonic, stomachic and alterative. Improves appetite and gives general tone to the body. Specially suitable in pregnancy.

### Galitakusthari Rasa.

Bhav Prakash.

Dose, 1 to 4 pills, to be taken twice a day after meals with milk or water. Each pill contains 1/22 gr. nux vomica. Chief ingredients are Kajjali, Tamra Bhasma, Loha Bhasma, Shilajatu, Vishtinduka, Abhrak Bhasma, etc. Tonic, alterative and stimulant. Recommended in Shastras for leprosy.

### Gulma Kalanal Rasa.

Rasa Sar. Samgraha.

Dose, 1 to 4 pills with milk, every morning. Chief ingredients are Kajjali, Loha Bhasma, Tamra Bhasma, Haratal, Yavakshara, and other stomachic tonic drugs. Tonic, stomachic, antiperiodic and alterative. Specially suitable for bowel complaints ; gives tone to the bowels and cures flatulent diarrhœa, feverishness and hyperacidity.

### Grahani Kapat Rasa.

Nighant Part II.

Dose 1 to 4 pills, to be taken three times a day with whey. Each pill contains 1/10 gr. Cannabis Indica. Chief ingredients are Kajjali, Abhrak Bhasma, Visha, Haritaki, Vacha. Alterative, astringent, anodyne. Specially suitable in sprue. Also useful in chronic diarrhœa.

### Grahani Vajra Kapat Rasa.

Rasa Sar Samgraha.

Dose, 1 to 4 pills, three times a day with whey. Antacid, alterative. Cures hyperacidity and relieves pain, discomfort and distention of the bowels. Specially suitable in sprue.

**Chakri Rasa.**

**Bhai. Ratna**

**Dose, 1 to 2 pills, two times a day after food. Each pill contains 1/9 gr. aconite, 1/9 gr. Datura folia, ⅓ gr. orpiment, 1/36 gr. croton seeds. Chief ingredients are Kajjali, aconite, Datura leaves, maricha, orpiment and croton seeds. Very useful in the treatment of malaria, chlorosis, diabetes, psoriasis, chronic eczema and other chronic skin affections.**

**For contra-indications, see Sanjivani Guti.**

**Chaturmukh Rasa.**

Rasa Sar. Samgraha.

**Dose 1 to 4 pills, to be taken twice a day after meals. Chief ingredients are Kajjali, Loha Bhasma, Abhrak Bhasma and Suvarna Bhasma. Tonic and hæmatinic. Useful in phthisis, cough, anæmia, asthma, epilepsy and various other skin diseases.**

**Chandrakala Rasa.**

Yoga Ratna.

Dose, 1 to 4 pills, to be taken three times a day. Chief ingredients are Ela, Karpura, Manashila, Amalaka, Jatiphala, Nagapushpa, Kajjali, Banga Bhasma, Loha Bhasma. Sedative, antispasmodic. Recommended in Shastras for internal hæmorrhages, such as hæmoptysis, hemetemesis, melæna, etc. Also in hæmaturia, dysuria, gleet and other urinary affections. For melæna, this should be given with whey and for urinary affections, with Mootra-virechan Quath.

**Jalodarari Rasa.**

Rasa Sara Samgraha.

**Dose, 1 to 3 pills, to be taken with milk. Each pill contains 1/3 gr. croton seeds. Other ingredients are Tamra Bhasma, Darvi and pipers. Powerful cathartic. Useful in ascites and dropsy. Produces copious stools.**

## RASAS (Mercurial Preparations).

Contra-indicated in feeble subjects, having organic obstruction or in inflammatory conditions of the stomach and intestines.

### Jatifaladya Gutika.

Rasa Sar Samgraha.

Dose, 1 to 4 pills to be taken three times a day with whey or water. Each pill contains 1/22 gr. aconite. Chief ingredients are Kajjali, Jatiphala Mocharasa, Visha, Maricha, Jiraka and acon Anodyne, astringent, diaphoretic. Useful in dysentery, acute or chronic diarrhœa, colic and other bowel complaints.

### Jwar Murari Rasa.

Yoga Ratna.

Dose, 1 to 4 pills to be taken three times a day with water. Each pill contains 1/12 gr. aconite. Chief ingredients are Kajjali, Naga Bhasma, Loha Bhasma, Abhraka Bhasma, Tamra Bhasma. Diaphoretic, Tonic. Reduces feverishness. Useful in pneumonia, tonsilitis. croup, bronchitis, asthma, etc.

For contra-indications, see Sanjivani Guti.

### Tamra Parpati.

Nighant Part II.

Dose, 1 to 2 grs. to be taken twice a day with Ghee or honey. Useful in cough, asthma, and other chest affections. Effects and uses, same as Tamra Bhasma..

### Tripur Bhairav Rasa.

Bhav Prakash.

Dose, 2 to 6 pills, to be given every 3 hours, until fever subsides. Not more than 20 pills to be given during 24 hours. Each pill contains 1/18 gr. aconite. Chief ingredients are aconite, Tamra Bhasma, Trikatu, Rasa Sindura, etc. Anodyne, antiphlogistic, antipyretic and diaphoretic. Most valuable in high fever and all local acute inflammations, such as those of pneumonia, eruptive fevers, erysipelas, tonsilitis and painful neuralgic affections.

For contra indications, see Sanjivani Guti.

### Tribhuvan Keerti Rasa.

Yoga Ratna.

Dose, 2 to 6 pills, to be given every two hours, until fever subsides. Not to be given more than 24 pills in 24 hours. Each pill contains 1-24 gr. aconite. Chief ingredients are Rasasindura, aconite, Trikatu, Pippali Moola, etc. Anodyne, antipyretic, and diaphoretic. Most useful in high fever and all local acute inflammations, such as those of pneumonia, eruptive fevers, erysipelas, tonsilitis and painful neuralgic affections.

For contra-indications, see Sanjivani Guti.

### Trailokya Chintamani Rasa.

Yoga Ratna.

Dose, 1 to 3 pills, three times a day. Each pill contains 1/24 gr. aconite. Chief ingredients are Kajjali, Heerak (Diamond) Bhasma, Suvarna Bhasma, Raupya Bhasma, Tamra Bhasma, Abhraka Bhasma, Mukta Bhasma, Praval Bhasma, Vaikrant Bhasma, Haritala, Manashila and aconite. Useful in gastric disorders, general debility, cough, asthma, phthisis, diarrhœa, colic, indigestion, anæmia, sexual debility, etc.

For contra-indications, see Sanjivani Guti.

### Devkusumadi Rasa.

Bhav Prakash.

Dose, 1 to 4 pills, to be given three times a day. Each pill contains 1/32 gr. Mercuric Chloride. Chief ingredients are Lavanga, Chandana, Saffron and Mercuric Chloride. The best remedy for syphilitic affections. Also useful in syphilitic and non-syphilitic skin affections.

## RASAS (Mercurial Preparations).

### Naracha Rasa.

Sha. M. Ch. XII.

Dose, 1 to 3, when desired. Each pill contains 1/3 gr. croton seeds. Chief ingredients are Kajjali, croton seeds, Trikatu, etc. Powerful purgative. Useful in obstinate constipation, cirrhosis, ascites, dropsy, etc.

Contra-indicated in feeble subjects; where there is organic obstruction, or in inflammatory conditions of the stomach and intestines.

### Narayan Jwarankusha.

Yoga Ratna.

Dose, 1 to 4 pills, to be taken three times a day after food. Each pill contains 1/120 gr. arsenic, and 1/18 gr. aconite. Chief ingredients are Arsenic, aconite, Kajjali, Haritala, Trikatu, etc. Should not be continued uninterruptedly for more than one month.

For contra indications, see Sanjivani Guti.

Very useful in the treatment of malaria, chlorosis, anæmia, diabetes, psoriasis, chronic eczema, etc.

### Nityanand Rasa.

Rasa Sar. Samgraha.

Dose, 1 to 4 pills to be taken three times a day with cold water. Each pill contains 1/50 gr. copper sulphate. Chief ingredients are Kajjali, Tamra Bhasma, Banga Bhasma, Haritala, Tuttha, Loha Bhasma, 5 salts and other stomachics. Tonic, alterative. Useful in elephantiasis.

### Panch Vakra Rasa.

Sha. M., Ch. XII.

Dose, 1 to 4 pills to be taken every 3 hours—not more than 16 in a day. Each pill contains 1/12 gr. aconite. Chief ingredients are Kajjali, aconite, Maricha, Pippali, etc. Antipyretic, diaphoretic, anodyne. Specially useful in fevers, and all local and acute inflammations, such as those of pneumonia, erysipelas, tonsilitis and painful neuralgic affections.

**Panchamrit Parpati. No. 1.**

Nighant Part II.

Dose, 2 to 8 grains, to be taken twice a day with Pippali (Piper Longum) powder. Most efficacious medicine for sprue and chronic diarrhœa.

**Panchamrit Parpati. No 2.**

Nighant Part II.

Dose and use same as above.

**Pasnupatastra Rasa.**

Vaid. Sar. Samgraha

Dose, 1 to 4 pills, twice a day with sugar and honey. Specially suitable in chronic ulcers, carbuncle, erysipelas, scrofula, goitre, etc.

Chief ingredients are Rasasindura, Loha Bhasma, Suvarna Bhasma, Abhraka Bhasma, Raupya Bhasma, Praval-Makshika-Mukta-Naag and Bang Bhasmas, &c.

**Pittabhanji Rasa.**

Dose 2 to 6 grains to be taken three hours before the usual time of attack of malarial fever, with sugar or piper longum (Krishna). Specially useful for pregnant women in fever attacks.

**Pradararipoo Rasa.**

Vaid. Sar Samgraha.

Dose, 1 to 4 pills three times a day with rice water. Chief ingredients are Kajjali, Naag Bhasma, Rasanjana and Lodhra. Tonic, astringent, alterative. Gives tone to the female reproductive organs and cures leucorrhœa and other female complaints. Is also useful in chronic diarrhœa.

**Brihat Chandrodaya Makardhwaj. 6 gr. pill.**

Bhaishaj. R. Dhwajbhang.

Dose, 1 to 4 pills, to be taken twice a day with milk. These pills are prepared by mixing the anupan with Chandrodaya Rasa as prescribed in Bhaishajya Ratnavali. Tonic, stimulant. Said to be highly efficacious in sexual debility.

### Mahajwarankusha Rasa.

Sha. M., Ch. XII.

Each pill contains 1 gr. Dattura seeds and 1 gr. aconite. Dose, 1 to 4 pills, as directed by the physician, to be taken every three hours with sugar, during relapse of fever. Chief ingredients are Kajjali, aconite, Dalttura seeds and Hemaksheera. Extensively used to check attacks of malarial fever.

For contra indications see Sanjivani Guti.

### Maha Mrityunjaya Rasa.

Rasa Sar. Samgraha. Pliha.

Each pill contains 1/20 grs. Tuttha (Copper Sulphate). Chief ingredients are Kajjali, Loha Bhasma, Abhraka Bhasma, Tamra Bhasma, Manashila, Yavakshara, Swarjikakshara, etc. Dose, 1 to 4 pills to be taken 3 times a day with water or Toolasi Rasa. Nervine tonic. Useful in fever. Cures fever without its bad effect of causing subsequent debility. Is also used in epilepsy and diarrhœa.

### Maha Mrityunjaya Loha.

Bhaishajya Ratna Pliha-Yakrit

Dose, 1 to 4 pills twice a day after meals. Chief ingredients are Kajjali, Abhraka Bhasma, Loha Bhasma, Tamra Bhasma, Yavakshara, Swarjika, Manashila, Haritala, Tuttha, etc. Alterative, tonic, diaphoretic. Useful in diseases of spleen, in cirrhosis, jaundice, hepatic colic, asthma and headache. This can be given with advantage in malaria with enlargement of spleen.

### Mahalaxmivilas Rasa.

Yoga Ratna Rajyakshma.

Dose 1 to 4 pills, three times a day with milk. Tonic, alterative, hæmatinic. Useful in phthisis, anæmia, dropsy, coryza, general debility, and sexual debility.

### Mrigank Vatika.

Bhaishajya Ratna.

Dose, 1 to 4 pills, with milk, twice a day after meals. Chief ingredients are Kajjali, Loha Bhasma, Abhrak Bhasma, Trikatu, Trifala, Pippali, etc. Tonic, hæmatinic, alterative. Largely used in phthisis.

### Mrityunjaya Rasa.

Rasendra Sar Sang. Jwar.

Dose, 1 to 3 pills three times a day with water. Each pill contains 1/6 gr. aconite. Chief ingredients are Kajjali, aconite, Tankana, etc. Diaphoretic, antipyretic, anodyne and diuretic. Most useful in fever, nasal catarrh, sore throat, neuralgia, acute gout and all acute inflammations of pneumonia, erysipelas, tonsilitis, and painful neuralgic affections.

For contra indications see Sanjivani Guti.

### Mehamudgara Rasa.

Bhaishajya Ratna. Prameha.

Dose, 1 to 4 pills to be taken twice a day after meals. Chief ingredients are Loha Bhasma, Rasanjana, Darvi, Gokshura, Bilva, Guggulu, etc. Tonic, antiperiodic, demulcent, diuretic, alterative. Useful in cases of spermatorrhœa, and other disorders of the urinary tract.

## RASAS (Mercurial Preparations.)

### 1 Yograj Guggulu (Maha).

Sha. M., Ch. VII.

Dose, 1 to 4 pills three times a day. Chief ingredients are Guggulu, Triphala, Banga Bhasma, Raupya Bhasma, Naga Bhasma, Loha Bhasma, Abhrak Bhasma, Mandura Bhasma, Rasa Sindura, etc. Alterative, tonic. Useful in synovitis, paraplagia, sciatica, hemiplegia and other nervous affections. It is also useful in anæmia, chlorosis, heart affection and scrofula.

### Ratnagiri Rasa. No. 2.

Dose, 2 to 6 grs. to be taken every three hours until fever subsides, with Dhanyak (Coriander) water. Alterative, diaphoretic. Most valuable in fevers, causes no weakness. As this preparation does not contain aconite, it can safely be given where aconite is contra indicated.

### Rasendra Gutika.

Bhaishajya Ratna.

Dose, 1 to 4 twice a day with milk or water. Chief ingredients are Loha Bhasma, Abhrak Bhasma, Kajjali, Praval Bhasma and Kharpar. Tonic, hæmatinic, alterative. Cures cough, asthma and hoarseness of voice, and other chest affections. Invigorates the body and is useful in anæmia, chlorosis, etc..

### Ramban Rasa.

Vai. Sar. Sangraha.

Dose, 1 to 4 pills, with Ghee, three times a day after meals. Each pill contains 1/64 gr. arsenic. Chief ingredients are Haritala, Hingula, Gandhaka, etc. Tonic, antiperiodic. This is valuable in malaria when Quinine is not tolerated. It is also useful in chronic skin diseases, e.g. eczema, psoriasis, lichen, pemphigus, etc. It gives good results in neuralgia, chronic rheumatism, gout, chronic nasal catarrh, cardiac weakness, scrofula, asthma, etc.

This medicine should not be continuously taken for more than 15 days.

**Laxminarayan Rasa.**

Yoga Ratna.

Dose, 1 to 3 pills every three hours. No more than 20 pills to be given during 24 hours. Each pill contains 1/20 gr. aconite. Chief ingredients are Abhrak Bhasma, Rasasindura, Vatsanabha, Katuki, Kutajatwak, etc., Anodyne, antiphlogistic, antipyretic and diaphoretic. Very useful in convulsions, hemicrania, neuralgia, etc.

For contra indications, see Sanjivani Guti.

**Laxmivilas Rasa.**

Rasasar Samgraha, Vajikaran.

Dose, 1 to 4 pills twice a day, wrapped in betel leaves followed by milk. Chief ingredients are Abhrak Bhasma, Kajjali, Camphor, Dattura seeds, cannabis Indica, and other nutritive tonics. Tonic, aphrodisiac, anodyne, hypnotic. Specially prepared for sexual debility, also useful in mania, spasmodic coughs, phthisis, asthma, acute neuralgia, dysmenorrhea and tetanus. Removes general debility and strengthens the body.

**Loknath Rasa.**

Bhai Ratna. Pliha.

Dose, 1 to 4 pills to be taken three times a day with honey and Pippali (piper longum) followed by milk. Chief ingredients are Kajjali, Abhrak Bhasma, Loha Bhasma, Tamra Bhasma. Useful in diseases of liver, dropsy, anæmia, jaundice, weakness subsequent to an attack of fever, etc

**Loha Parpati.**

Dose, 2 to 6 grains with honey, twice a day after meals. Useful in sprue, chronic diarrhœa, dysentery and anæmia.

## RASAS (Mercurial Preparations.)

### Vadvanal Rasa,

Rasasar Samgraha.

Dose, 1 to 4 tablets three times a day. Chief ingredients are Kajjali, Panch Lavana, Yavakshar, Swarjikakshar and Tankana. Stomachic, antacid, diuretic and carminative. Removes hyperacidity, flatulence, tympanitis, indigestion, dyspepsia. It is also useful in gout and gonorrhoea.

### Vasant Kusumakar Rasa.

Bhaish Ratna. Bahumootra.

Dose, 1 to 4 pills, three times a day with milk. Chief ingredients are Vaikrant Bhasma, Suvarna Bhasma, Abhrak Bhasma, Mukta Bhasma, Praval Bhasma, Bang Bhasma and Rasa Bhasma. Useful in diabetes insipidus and other urinary affections, also in sexual debility, phthisis, asthma and general weakness.

### (Suvarna) Vasant Malati No. 2.

Dose, 2 to 8 grs. twice a day with piper longum and honey followed by milk. Extensively used in phthisis, cough. Removes debility and promotes appetite.

### Vasant Malati. No. 3.

Dose, 2 to 8 grs. to be taken with piper longum and honey followed by milk, three times during the day. Uses and effect same as above.

### Vataraktantak Rasa.

Rasasar Samgraha. Vatrakta.

Dose, 1 to 4 pills, twice a day with Nimbadi quath. Chief ingredients are Kajjali, Loha Bhasma Manashila, Haritala, Abhrak Bhasma, Shilajatu, Guggulu, etc. Alterative, tonic ; useful in rheumatism and gouty affections, hemiplegia, paraplegia, facial paralysis and other paralytic affections.

## Vatari Rasa. 2 gr. pill.

Bhav Prakash. Vatrog.

Dose, 1 to 4 pills to be taken three times a day with Rasnadi quath. Chief ingredients are Kajjali, Triphala, Chitraka and Guggulu. Alterative, tonic. Useful in orchitis, sciatica, paralysis agitans, paralysis facial, paraplegia, hemiplegia and other nervous and paralytic affections.

## Vishva Tap Haran Rasa.

Nighant Part II.

Dose, 1 to 4 pills with water when desired. Each pill contains 1/9 gr. nux vomica and as much croton seeds. Chief ingredients are Kajjali, Tamra Bhasma, Nux vomica and croton seeds. Purgative, diaphoretic and stimulant. Useful in chronic constipation, fever, chronic paralytic affections.

## Shankha Vati.

Nighant Part II.

Dose, 1 to 4 tablets when necessary, but not more than 10 tablets in 24 hours. Each tablet contains 1/10 grs. aconite. Chief ingredients are Shankh Bhasma, Chinchakshara, 5 salts, Trikatu, Kajjali and aconite. Sedative, stomachic. Useful in indigestion, tympanitis. Gives immediate relief in intestinal colic.

## Shwasakuthara Rasa.

Bhav Prakash.

Dose, 1 to 4 pills, with water when desired. Each pill contains 1/15 gr. aconite. Chief ingredients are Kajjali, aconite, Manashila, Maricha and Trikatu. Sedative, gastric, stimulant, diaphoretic. Very efficacious in asthma, fevers, and all local acute inflammations, such as those of pneumonia, erysipelas, tonsilitis and painful neuralgic affections.

### Shwas Chintamani Rasa.

Bhaishajya. Hicca

Dose, 1 to 4 pills to be taken three times a day with honey and Bibhitak Churna. Chief ingredients are Loha Bhasma, Gandhaka, Abhrak Bhasma, Kajjali, Makshika, Mukta and Suvarna Bhasmas. Alterative, tonic. Useful in cough, asthma, phthisis, anæmia, chlorosis. general debility, etc.

### Sarwanga Sundara Rasa.

Rasasar Samgraha.

Dose, 1 to 4 pills to be taken three-times a day with Shunthi quath or hot water. Chief ingredients are Kajjali, Tamra Bhasma, Manashila, Makshika, Haritala, Raupya Bhasma, Suvarna Bhasma, Banga Bhasma, Loha Bhasma, Abhraka Bhasma. Alterative, sedative. Useful in indigestion and intestinal colic, phthisis, asthma and general debility.

### Sarveshwar Parpati.

Dose, 2 to 6 grs. to be taken twice a day with Ghee, honey or butter. Useful in phthisis, internal abscess, and chronic fevers.

### Siddha Lakshmivilas Rasa.

Vaidya Sar Samgraha.

Dose 1 to 4 pills, to be taken three times a day with milk. Chief ingredients are Rasa Bhasma, Suvarna Bhasma, Raupya Bhasma, Tamra Bhasma, Loha Bhasma, Mandura Bhasma, Banga Bhasma, Naga Bhasma, Mukta Bhasma, Praval Bhasma. Alterative, tonic, hæmatinic. Useful in phthisis, anæmia, cough, asthma and diabetes.

### Suvarna Parpati.

Dose, 2 to 6 grs. to be taken twice a day with Ghee or Butter. Useful in phthisis, general debility, weakness of memory, etc.

### Suta Shekhara Rasa.

Yoga Ratna. Amlapitta.

Dose, 1 to 4 pills, twice a day with water or cocoanut water. Each pill contains 1/17 gr. aconite and 1/17 gr. Dattura seeds. Chief ingredients are Suvarna Bhasma, Shankha Bhasma, aconite, Dattura seeds, Bilvapeshika, etc. Useful in hyper-acidity, vomiting, indigestion, colic, cough, asthma, diarrhœa, dysentery, giddiness and convulsions.

For contra indications, see Sanjivani Gutika.

### Sootikabharan Rasa.

Yoga Ratna. Vatroaga.

Dose, 1 to 4 pills, to be taken with water or Devdarvadi quath, twice a day. Chief ingredients are Suvarna Bhasma, Raupya Bhasma, Tamra Bhasma, Praval Bhasma, Kajjali, Abhrak Bhasma, Haritala, Manashila. Useful in tetanus, and puerperal diseases.

### Smriti Sagar Rasa.

Yoga Ratna Apasmar.

Dose, 1 to 4 pills, to be taken twice a day with Brahmi Ghrita followed by milk. Alterative, tonic. Chief ingredients are Kajjali, Haital, Manashila and Tamra Bhasma. Specially suitable for epilepsy, mania and weakness of memory.

## BHASMAS.

All the Bhasmas mentioned below are manufactured at the Jamnagar Rasa Shala, which is the oldest Rasashala in the Bombay Presidency, having been established in A.D. 1865. The Rasa Shala enjoys the confidence of its constituents for its preparations, which are prepared strictly according to Shastras. People, therefore, prefer to buy Bhasmas made by the Jamnagar Rasa Shala in preference to many other similar but cheaper preparations of other frms.

**Abhrak Bhasma** (Sahasra Puti).

Sha. M. Ch. XII.

Dose, 2 to 6 grs, to be taken twice with honey. Useful in phthisis, and debility of old age; gives strength to the body.

**Abhrak Bhasma** (Shata Puti).

Dose and use, same as above.

**Abhrak Bhasma** (with Amritikaran).

Dose and use, same

**Chandrodaya No. 1.** (Suvarna Ghatit Makardhwaj) Bhai Ratna. Rs. 75 0 0

Dose, 2 to 6 grs. to be taken twice a day with Chandrodaya Anupan and honey, followed by milk. Diet:—Oil and capsicum to be avoided. Most popular remedy in sexual debility.

**Chandrodaya No. 2.**

Dose, use, and diet restrictions same as above.

**Jasata Bhasma.**

Sha. M. Ch. XI.

Dose 2 to 6 grs. twice a day with honey or Ghee. Useful in internal hæmorrhages and urinary disorders.

**Tamra Bhasma.**

Sha. M. Ch. XI.

Dose 1 to 2 grs. to be taken twice a day with honey or Ghee. Useful in cough and asthma.

**Naag Bhasma.**

Sha. M Ch. XI.

Dose, 2 to 12 grs. to be taken twice a day with butter or Ghee. Oil, pungent spices and acid fruits to be strictly avoided. Removes urinary disorders and general debility.

**Praval Bhasma.**

Sha. M. Ch. XI.

Dose 3 to 12 grs. to be taken twice a day after food. Useful in scrofulous affections. carbuncle, spermatorrhœa, cough, phthisis, &c.

**Praval Panchamrit Bhasma.**

Yoga Ratnakar, Gulmaroag.

Does 2 to 6 grs. twice a day with honey. Chief ingredients are Praval Bhasma, Mukta Bhasma, Shankha Bhasma, Shukti Bhasma, Varatika Bhasma. Useful in general debility, especially that of tuberculosis, cough, tympanitis, carbuncle, spermatorrhœa and scrofulous affections.

**Banga Bhasma.**

Sha. M. Ch. XI.

Dose, 2 to 6 grs. to be taken twice a day with honey or butter. Useful in urinary disorders and general debility.

**Mandura Bhasma.**

Sha. M. Ch. XI.

Dose 2 to 16 grs. twice a day with butter or honey, after food. Useful in anæmia, chlorosis, general debility, sexual debility. Specially efficacious in pale and rickety children used to eat earth.

### Makshik Bhasma.

Sha. M. Ch. XI.

Dose 2 to 12 grs. to be taken twice a day with honey, after meals. Useful in anæmia, chlorosis, heart affections, scrofula and general debility.

### Mukta Bhasma.

Sha. M. Ch. XI.

Dose 2 to 6 grs. to be taken twice a day with honey. Useful in general debility, cough, phthisis and asthma.

### Raupya Bhasma.

Sha. M. Ch. XI.

Dose, 2 to 6 grs. to be taken twice a day with Ghee or honey. Useful in general debility.

### Loha Bhasma, No. 1.

Sha. M. Ch. XI.

Dose 1 to 5 grs. to be taken twice a day with honey, after meals. Tonic, hæmatinic. Useful in anæmia, chlorosis, delirium, erysipelatous inflammations, Bright's disease, heart affections, scrofula, phthisis, general debility and sexual debility.

### Loha Bhasma No. 2.

Dose, 2 to 6 grs. to be taken in the morning with Ghee or butter followed by milk. Tonic, hæmatinic. Improves blood, gives strength, cures anæmia, and is useful in all conditions of debility.

## Shankh Bhasma.

Dose, 2 to 4 grs, to be taken with whey, when desired. Useful in tympanitis, flatulence, colic, &c.

## Shouktik Bhasma.

Dose, 2 to 4 grs. to be taken twice a day, with milk or rice water. Useful in hæmorrhages, pulmonary or intestinal, hyper-acidity, giddiness.

## Suvarna Bhasma.

Sha. M. Ch. XI.

Dose 2 to 6 grs. to be taken twice a day with butter or honey. Useful in phthisis, strengthens memory and removes general debility.

## ASAVA AND ARISHTA.

**Amritarisht.** Bhai Ratna.

Dose ½ to 2 tolas, twice a day after meals. Chief ingredients are Gudoochi, Shatavari, Parpat, Saptaparna, Katuki, &c. Bitter tonic and stimulant. Specially useful in chronic fevers, removes after-debility and improves appetite.

**Oosheera Asava.**

Bhai Ratna.

Dose ½ to 2 tolas, twice a day after meals. Chief ingredients are Valaka, Padma, Lodhra, Manjistha, Parpat, Mochrasa, Draksha, Dhatakipushpa, etc. Alterative, tonic, astringent. Useful in intestinal and pulmonary hæmorrhages, chronic diarrhœa.

**Kanaka Asava.**

Bhaishajya Ratnavali.

Dose ½ to 2 tolas, twice after meals. Chief ingredients are Kanaka, Vasa, Yastimadhu, Pippali, Dhatakipushpa and Draksha. Demulcent, expectorant, antispasmodic and anodyne. Useful in cough. asthma, phthisis.

**Kootaja Arista.**

Bhaishajya Ratnavali.

Dose ½ to 2 tolas, twice after meals. Chief ingredients are Kootajatwak, Draksha, Madhuka Pushpa, Kashmari, Dhatakipushpa, &c. Astringent, stimulant and antiperiodic. Efficacious in chronic diarrhœa, sprue, dysentery and long continued fevers.

**Kumari Asava.**

Gad Nigraha.

..ose ½ to 2 tolas, twice after meals. Chief in gredients are Kumari, Dashamoola, Pushkarmoola,

Dhanvayasa, Chitraka, Draksha, Dhataki Pushpa. This preparation contains about 70 drugs in all. Stimulant, laxative, alterative. Useful in cough, asthma, piles, tympanitis, colic, chronic constipation, etc.

### Chavika Asava.

Gad Nigraha.

Dose ½ to 2 tolas, to be taken as directed. Chief ingredients are Chavya, Chitraka, Pushkarmoola, Jeeraka. Stimulant. Useful in nasal catarrh, phthisis, cough, flatulence.

### Dashamoola Asava.

Gad Nigraha.

Dose ½ to 2 tolas, twice a day after meals. Chief ingredients are Dashamoola, Pushkar Moola, Dhanvayasa, Gudoochi, Lodhra, Amalaki, Haritaki, Draksha, Dhataki Pushpa, &c. Stimulant, alterative and bitter tonic. Useful in cough, piles, anorexia, alcoholism, asthma, vomiting.

### Draksha Asava.

Sha. M. Ch. X.

Dose ½ to 2 tolas, to be taken twice a day after meals or when desired. Chief ingredients are Draksha, Dhataki Pushpa and sugar. Stimulant, (especially cardiac), antipyretie, diuretic and diaphoretic. Useful in chronic wasting diseases, such as phthisis, insomnia of old people, loss of appetite, sudden fainting, cough. Maintains strength in acute diseases characterised by excessive debility.

### Pippali Arishta.

Gad Nigraha.

Dose ½ to 2 tolas as directed. Chief ingredients are Pippali, Lodhra, Maricha, Patha, Draksha, &c. Stimulant. Useful in piles, cough, anorexia, asthma, etc.

## ASAVA AND ARISHTA.

### Rohitaka Asava.

Dose ½ to 2 tolas, to be taken twice a day after meals. Chief ingredients are Rohitaka, Triphala, Dhataki Pushpa, etc. Tonic, alterative. Useful in diseases of spleen and liver.

### Loha Asava.

Bhaishajya Ratnavali.

Dose ½ to 2 tolas, to be taken as directed. Chief ingredients are Loha, Trikatu, Trifala, Vidanga, &c. Tonic, alterative. Useful in anæmia, dropsy and diseases of spleen.

# MISCELLANEOUS PREPARATIONS

### Gudoochi Satva.

This is obtained from Gudoochi. Dose 6 to 24 grs. to be taken with sugar and milk. Useful in feverishness, general debility, headache and urinary disorders.

### Apamarga Kshar.

Dose 2 to 4 grs. to be taken with honey. This Kshar is largely used in ascites, dropsy, cutaneous affections and enlargement of glands. It is also used to loosen expectoration in cough. Used also externally for application in dog bites and scorpion bites.

### Chincha Kshar.

Dose 4 to 10 grs. to be taken with honey. Alkaline. Useful in acidity of urine, gonorrhœa, acidity of stomach, colic and rheumatism.

### Yava Kshar.

Dose 5 to 30 grs. to be taken thrice a day with water. Antacid, antilithic, diuretic. Useful in dyspepsia, gout, acute gonorrhœa, bronchitis, pneumonia influenza, calculi renal.

### Vajra Kshar.

Rasendra Sar Samgraha

Dose 2 to 8 grs: to be taken before meals with warm water or ghee. Chief ingredients are four salts and three ksharas. Gastric stimulant, antacid. Useful in tympanitis, colic, dyspepsia, indigestion, hyperacidity.

### Shankha Drava.

Yoga Ratnaker.

Dose 2 to 5 drops diluted in 1 oz. of water or Shunthi Quath. Chief ingredients are Navasagar, Yavakshâra, Swarjika, Phatika, Kasisa and Soura kshar. Cholagogue and gastric tonic. Useful in tropical enlargement and chronic congestion of the liver, biliousness, oxaluria and in torpid conditions of the stomach and catarrhal jaundice, etc.

### Nayana Amrita.

Yoga Ratnaker.

To be applied in the eyes. Is a good collyrium. Keeps the eyes cool. When used continuously, restores sight.

## SANSKRIT AND LATIN EQUIVALENTS.

| Sanskrit. | Latin. |
|---|---|
| Abhaya .. | .. Terminalia Chebula. |
| Agaru .. | .. Aquilaria Agallocha. |
| Agnimanth | .. Premna Integrifolia |
| Ajamoda .. | .. Carum Roxburghianam. |
| Akarkarabh | .. Anacyclus Pyrethrum. |
| Amalaka .. | .. Phyllanthus Emblica. |
| Amlavetasa. | .. Rumex Vesicarius. |
| Amrasthi .. | .. Mango-stone. |
| Amrita. .. | .. Tinospora Cordifolia. |
| Apamarga . | .. Achyranthes Aspera. |
| Arani .. | .. Premna Integrifolia. |
| Arka .. | .. Calotropis Procera. |
| Ashoka .. | .. Joneshia Ashoka. |
| Ashmabheda | .. Coleus Aromaticus. |
| Ashwagandha | .. Withania Somnifera. |
| Ashwatha .. | .. Ficus Religiosa. |
| Atibala .. | .. Abutilon Indicum. |
| Avalguja .. | .. Psoralea Corylifolia. |
| Babbhul .. | .. Acacia Arabica. |
| Bakuchi .. | .. Psoralea Corylifolia. |
| Bhallataka . | .. Semecarpus Anacardium. |
| Bhringaraj . | .. Eclipta Alba. |
| Bibhitaka .. | .. Terminalia Belerica. |
| Bida Lavan | .. Vit salt. |
| Bilva .. | .. Aegle Marmelos. |
| Brahmi .. | .. Hydrocotyle Asiatica. |
| Brihati .. | .. Solanum Indicum. |
| Chakramarda | .. Cassia Tora. |
| Chandana .. | .. Santanum Album. |
| Changeri .. | .. Oxalis Corniculata. |
| Chaturjata . | .. Twak, Tamalpatra, Ela and Nagpushpa. |
| Chavya .. | .. Piper Chaba. |
| Chincha .. | .. Tamarindus Indica. |
| Chitraka . | .. Plumbago Zeylanica. |
| Chopchini .. | .. Smilex Glabra. |
| Dadima .. | .. Punica Granatum. |
| Danti .. | .. Croton Tiglium. |

## SANSKRIT AND LATIN EQUIVALENTS.

| Sanskrit. | Latin. |
|---|---|
| Darbha .. | .. Eragrostis Cynosuroides. |
| Darvi .. | .. Berberis Aristata. |
| Deodara .. | .. Cedrus Deodara. |
| Dhanvayasa | .. Fagonia Arabica. |
| Dhanyaka . | .. Coriandrum Sativum. |
| Dhataki .. | .. Woodfordia Floribunda. |
| Dhustura .. | .. Datura Stramonium. |
| Draksha .. | .. Vitis Vinifera. |
| Ela . .. | .. Elettaria Cardamomum. |
| Eliyaka .. | .. Alœs. |
| Gangeruki | .. Grewia Populifolia. |
| Gandhaka . | .. Sulphur. |
| Gokshuraka | .. Tribulus Terrestris. |
| Gooduchi .. | .. Tinospora Cordifolia. |
| Guggulu .. | .. Commiphora Mucal. |
| Gunja .. | .. Abrus Precatorius. |
| Haritaki .. | .. (See Abhaya.) |
| Hingupatri . | .. Peucedanum Grande. |
| Indrayava . | .. Holarrhena Antidysenterica. |
| Irimeda .. | .. Acacia Farnesiana. |
| Jambuasthi. | .. Jambulstone. |
| Jasat-pushpa | .. Zinc Oxide. |
| Jatiphala .. | .. Myristica Fragrans (fruit). |
| Jatipatri .. | .. " " (bark). |
| Jiraka .. | .. Cuminum Cyminum. |
| Jyotishmati | .. Celastrus Paniculata. |
| Kajjali .. | .. Mercury and Sulphur. |
| Kakubha .. | .. Terminalia Arjun. |
| Kanchanar . | .. Bauhinia Variegata. |
| Kankola .. | .. Piper Cubeba. |
| Kantkarika | .. Solanum Xanthocarpum. |
| Kapittha .. | .. Feronia Elephantum. |
| Karanja .. | .. Pongamia Glabra. |
| Karpasmoola. | .. Root of Gossypium. |
| Karpur .. | .. Camphor. |
| Kasisa .. | .. Sulphate of Iron. |
| Katphala .. | .. Mirica Nagi. |
| Katuki .. | .. Picrorrhiza Kurroa. |
| Katurohini . | .. " " |
| Keshara .. | .. Messua Ferea. |
| Kindaru .. | .. Boswellia Seretta. |
| Kirata .. | .. Swertia Chirata. |

| Sanskrit. | Latin. |
|---|---|
| Kirmani .. | .. Artemisia Maritima. |
| Kokilaksha | .. Hygrophila Spinosa. |
| Krishna lavana | .. Black salt. |
| Ksharas .. | .. Yavakshara & Swargika. |
| Kshwavak.. | .. Artemisia Sternutatoria. |
| Kuberaksha | .. Cæsalpinia Bonducella. |
| Kunkuma . | .. Saffron. |
| Kusha .. | .. Poa Cynosuroides. |
| Kustha .. | .. Saussurea Lappa. |
| Kutaj .. | .. Holarrhema Antidysenterica |
| Lajjalu .. | .. Mimosa Pudica. |
| Laksha .. | .. Tacharida Lacca. |
| Lashuna . | .. Alium Sativum. |
| Lavang .. | .. Eugenia Caryophyllata. |
| Lodhra .. | .. Symplocos Racemosa. |
| Madan .. | .. Randia Dumetorum. |
| Madhuka .. | .. Glycerrhiza Glabra. |
| Mahanimba. | .. Melia Azedarach. |
| Manashila . | .. Realgar. |
| Manjistha .. | .. Rubia Cordifolia. |
| Mansi .. | .. Nardostachys Jatamansi. |
| Maricha .. | .. Piper Nigrum. |
| Markandi .. | .. Senna. |
| Mocharasa.. | .. Bombax Malabaricum. |
| Moolaka .. | .. Raphanus Sativus. |
| Moorva .. | .. Clematis Triloba. |
| Moosali .. | .. Hypoxis Orchioides. |
| Mundi .. | .. Sphœranthus Indicus. |
| Musta .. | .. Cyperus Rotundus. |
| Nagpushpa | .. Messua Ferea. |
| Nakha .. | .. Nails. |
| Narikela .. | .. Cocoanut. |
| Navasagar.. | .. Chloride of Ammonia. |
| Nichula .. | .. Calamus Rotang. |
| Nimb .. | .. Melia Azadirachta. |
| Nirgundi .. | .. Vitex Negundo. |
| Padma .. | .. Nelumbium Speciosum. |
| Padmaka .. | .. Prunus Puddum. |
| Palasha .. | .. Butea Frondosa. |
| Panch lavana | .. Five salts. |
| Parada .. | .. Mercury. |
| Parpat .. | .. Rungia Repens. |

## SANSKRIT AND LATIN EQUIVALENTS.

| Sanskrit. | Latin. |
|---|---|
| Parsik Yavani | Artemisia Maritima. |
| Patala | Sterospermum Suaveolens. |
| Patha | Cissampelos Pareira. |
| Patol | Trichosanthes Dioica. |
| Phalamla | Garcina Indica. |
| Pippala | Ficus Religiosa. |
| Pippali | Piper Longum. |
| Pippalimoola | „ „ (Root) |
| Prastiparni | Craria Lagopoides. |
| Punarnava | Bœrhaavia Verticillata. |
| Raktchandana | Pterocarpus Santalinus. |
| Rasasindura | Mercurial Preparation. |
| Rasanjan | Extract of Berberis Aristata. |
| Raskarpura | Mercuric Chloride. |
| Rasna | Vanda Roxburghii. |
| Revanchi | Rheum Emodi. |
| Rohisha | Cymbopogon Martini. |
| Rohitaka | Tecoma Undulata. |
| Sahasara | Alœs. |
| Saindhava | Common salt. |
| Samudraphena | Sepia Officinalis. |
| Saptaparna | Alstonia Scholaris. |
| Sariva | Hemidesmus Indicus. |
| Sarshapa | Brassica Compestris. |
| Sauvarchala | Black salt. |
| Shakrayava | See Indrayava. |
| Shaliparni | Desmodium Gangenticum. |
| Shalmali | Bombax Malabaricum. |
| Shankh | Couchsheli. |
| Shankhpushpi | Convolvulus Mycrophyllus. |
| Sharpunkha | Tephrosia Purpurea. |
| Shatavari | Asparagus Racemosus. |
| Shathi | Curcuma Zedoaria. |
| Shatapusha | Fœniculum Vulgare. |
| Shigru | Moringa Pterygosperma. |
| Shirisha | Albizzia Lebbek. |
| Shiva | Terminalia Chebula. |
| Shringi | Rhus Succedanea. |
| Shunthi | Zingiber Officinale. |
| Shweta | Clitoria Ternatea. |
| Sidharthaka | Brassica Compestris. |
| Sinduvar | Vitex Negundo. |

| Sanskrit. | Latin. |
|---|---|
| Surana .. | .. Amorphophallus Campanulatus. |
| Surasa .. | .. Ocimum Sativum. |
| Surashtraja | .. Alum. |
| Suryakshara | .. Potassium Nitrate. |
| Swarjikakshara | .. Carbonate of Soda. |
| Syonaka .. | .. Oroxylum Indicum. |
| Tagar .. | .. Veleriana Wallichii. |
| Talisapatra | .. Pinus Webbiana. |
| Tamalpatra. | .. Cinnamomum Tamala. |
| Tankana .. | .. Borax. |
| Tankanamla | .. Boric acid. |
| Tiktajiraka | .. Vernonia Anthelmintica. |
| Tila . .. | .. Sesamum Indicum. |
| Tintidika .. | .. Tamarindus Indica. |
| Trapusha .. | .. Cucumis Sativus. |
| Trayanti .. | .. Ficus Heterophylla. |
| Trayamana | .. " " |
| Triphala .. | .. Three Myrobalans. |
| Trivrit .. | .. Operculina Turpethum. |
| Turushka .. | .. Liquidamber Orientalis. |
| Tuttha .. | .. Sulphate of Copper. |
| Twak .. | .. Cinnamomum Zeylanicum. |
| Udumbara.. | .. Ficus Glomerata. |
| Vacha .. | .. Acorus Calamus. |
| Valaka .. | .. Vetiveria Zizanioides. |
| Vanari .. | .. Mucuna Pruriens. |
| Vanshalochana | .. Bamboo Mana. |
| Varuna .. | .. Crataeva Religiosa. |
| Vasa. .. | .. Adhatoda Vasica. |
| Vidang .. | .. Embellia Ribes. |
| Vidari .. | .. Ipomœa Digitata. |
| Vijaya .. | .. Canabis Sativa |
| Virataru .. | .. Terminalia Arjun. |
| Visha .. | .. Aconitum Heterophyllum. |
| Vishatinduka | .. Nux Vomica. |
| Vridhadaraka | .. Argyreia Speciosa. |
| Yastimadhu | .. Glycerrhiza Glabra. |
| Yava .. | .. Hordeum Valgare. |
| Yavakshara | .. Carbonate of Potash. |
| Yavani .. | .. Carum Copticum. |

# DIET TABLES AND GENERAL DIRECTIONS.

The following directions for the diet and general regulation of life in certain diseases may be useful for reference. Such directions are, of course, only general and need careful modification for each case.

### ALBUMINURIA.

This dietary is especially intended for cases of Bright's disease, but with modification it may be used in cases of functional Albuminuria.

Allowed :—A liberal diet of readily assimilable food. Water of mung and other pulses, Roti of wheat, bajri and joar ; sago, rice, barley, green vegetables. e.g., onions, salads, mushrooms. cauliflower, turnips, milk, skim milk, whey, curdled milk, butter, ghee (in moderation), tea, coffee and cocoa (in moderation) ; sodawater, rice water, barley water.

Forbidden:—Sugar, ices, sweets, sweetballs and sweet foods generally : jellies, spiced foods, pickles. sauces, potatoes, peas, leaves. and thick pulses generally ; cheese, and every form of alcohol.

**General Directions :—**

1. A quiet life without worry or excitement.
2. A warm, dry house.
3. A warm, dry, equable climate.
4. Woollen clothing next the skin, night and day, all the year round.
5. Be sure that every possible care is taken to avoid catching cold.
6. Regular daily exercise, always stopping short of fatigue.
7. Maintain a free, regular action of the skin, kidneys, and bowels.
8. Hot vapour baths; tepid sponging with skin friction.
9. Avoid hot and cold baths; but warm baths may be taken.

### ANÆMIA.

Allowed :—A full generous diet containing relatively much albumin : pulses (unless there be dyspepsia, when the quantity should be very small) *i.e.* mung, tur, chana., etc., cereals e.g., wheat, bajri, joar, barley ; vegetables of all kinds ; all fruits, e.g., Amalaka, mango, banana ; milk, whey, cream, butter, ghee, oil, draksharasa. Salt in abundance. Fluids generally in abundance.

Forbidden :—Highly spiced foods, pickles, and all recooked foods.

**General Directions :—**

1. Abundant rest, especially in well ventilated rooms (sunny if possible), in the open air, and in the sunshine.

2. Moderate exercise, gradually increased, but always stopping short of fatigue. It should be taken preferably in several short walks rather than one long one. Patients suffering from anæmia, and invalid generally, often bear better the exercise taken after noon.

3. Regular daily skin friction, preceded by tepid sponging. Very few anæmia patients can take cold baths.

4. Be sure the teeth are in good condition.

5. Meals should be frequent, not at long intervals. Some nourishment, hot or cold milk, should be given half an hour before rising.

6. An insufficient quantity of fluid is a frequent cause of constipation in anæmia. It is a common experience that no remedies help the anæmia so long as the constipation lasts. Anæmia patients should be instructed to take not less than 3 or 3½ pints of fluid daily. By this, and other means, if necessary, any constipation must be relieved.

7. Anæmic children and women should be prevented from eating earth. If they have got that bad habit, they should be induced to take charcoal.

## CONSTIPATION.

Allowed:—Water of mung and dal, barley, wheat (choose the coarser flour of wheat for preparing roti and take roti in large quantities and with ghee), cabbage, mushrooms, salads (with abundant oil), and other vegetables if fresh or watery, onions, apples, figs, prunes, dates, oranges, grapes, bananas and tamarinds.

Forbidden:—Peas, beans, new potatoes, rice, nuts of all kinds; milk, except in small quantities; pickles, strong tea, cheese and pastry.

**General Directions :—**

1. Insist upon the patient taking a full quantity of fluid—for an adult at least 3 to 3½ pints daily.

2. This fluid may well include a tumblerful of water cold or hot immediately on getting out of bed.

3. Insist upon fruit or jam with farinaceous foods e.g., rice, and order every night or early morning a full quantity of such fruits as figs, baked apples, bananas, etc.

4. The body should be warmly clothed to avoid getting chilled, and the feet kept warm and dry by thick boots.

5. Tepid or cold bath followed by sharp frictions with a rough towel daily to secure a vigorous action of the skin.

6. Abdominal massage for ten minutes before rising every morning this (which can readily be done by the patients) followed by the cold or hot water on rising, is often sufficient to produce a speedy evacuation.

7. Regular exercise, especially of those kinds which bring abdominal muscles into play.

8. Insist upon the habit of regular hour every morning for the bowels to act whether there is desire or not.

# DIET TABLES.

## DIABETES.

Allowed :—Cream, butter, cheese ; mung and other pulses in small quantity ; green vegetables, cabbage, cauliflower, tomatoes, cucumber, mushrooms, all in great moderation ; oranges, lemons, nuts of all kinds except chestnuts ; pickles, oil, milk in great moderation, soda water.

Forbidden :—Sugar and starch in any form, rice, sago, vermicelly, arrowroot, cornflower, barley, potatoes, peas, pastry and puddings of all kinds, milk (except in small quantity) ; fruits of all kinds except those named (in moderation only).

**General Directions :—**

1. Regular daily exercise is extremely important, but fatigue should be avoided.
2. Flannel clothing next the skin always, most carefully guarding against catching cold.
3. A calm, equable, regular life without worry, excitement, or overwork
4. Regular action of the skin should be encouraged by tepid sponging, followed by skin friction by warm bathing and massage.

It is usually the better pratice gradually to lessen the carbo hydrate foods, until the sugar has disappeared, and afterwards tentatively replace them noting the effect of the each addition as a guide

## DIARRHŒA.

Allowed :—Cold milk (boiled for preference), plain, with lime water or barley water, whey, rice water ; mung water and rice, sago ; curry and rice ; tea.

**Note** :—In severe cases restrict the diet to whey and rice or whey alone.

Forbidden :—Thick pulses, green vegetables, acid fruits, potatoes, all hard foods, sweet balls.

**General Directions :—**

1. Warmth and absolute rest in bed.
2. Warm clothing, especially for the abdomen.
3. The food should be given in small quantities frequently.
4. During convalescence, the food should be increased cautiously.

## DYSPEPSIA.

The condition under which the digestion of food becomes inefficient or difficult are so many and have such widely varying causes, that no general diet rules can be drawn up. Those foods which are usually found digestible and indigestible are indicated below, but it is imperative that the diet be carefully chosen for each case.

Allowed :—Mung, wheat, bajri, joar in moderation ; rice, sago, potatoes, green vegetables generally in small quantity only ; fruits in small quantities ; milk, butter, ghee, in moderation ; oranges, prunes, hot or cold water, tea (not strong), whey, Draksharasa when necessary.

Forbidden :—Pastry and sweets; sauces, pickles and condiments; thick pulses; ice cream; all starchy and sugary foods, uncooked vegetables, acid unripe fruits; foods generally which leave a large residue or which are in their nature irritating.

**General Directions :—**

1. Be sure the teeth are sound and in such numbe and condition as to ensure complete mastication. One or more tender teeth which the owner dare not bite on, may alone lead to bolting of food and consequent indigestion. It is essential in every case to see not only that the teeth are sound, but that they are regularly used. Unused teeth usually get furred, coated and discoloured.
2. All food should be eaten slowly and completely masticated and little fluid taken with meals.
3. Meals should be taken at regular hours and when possible in pleasant company, without haste, and under conditions free from hurry, worry, or excitement. Each meal should, when possible, be preceded and followed by a short period of rest.
4. All foods should be so cooked and served as to stimulate appetite and digestion.
5. Where tea, coffee, tobacco, and stimulants are allowed, explicit instructions should be given as to the kind and quantity, and when and how they should be consumed. For example freshly-made tea and mild tobacco may be harmless, where strong tea and strong tobacco would be injurious.
6. Air, exercise, skin friction, suitable clothing, the avoidance of fatigue and care as to the bowels, are essentials in the rational treatment of dyspepsia.

## FEVERS.

Allowed :—Mung water, orange juice, kanji, Rab, etc. Generally milk is not allowed by Native Vaidyas for 7 days, but in alopathy it is allowed from the beginning of fever.

Forbidden :—Cold baths, exercise, ghee, pulses, sweets, heavy foods, generally all solids until after the crisis; in typhoid, solid food should not usually be given until after a week after the temperature becomes permanently normal.

## GOUT.

Allowed :—All fresh vegetables freely (with exceptions named), rice, sago, fresh ripe fruits (with exceptions named), wheat, bajri, joar, potatoes, salads, milk, milk puddings, lime-juice freely diluted, tea (not strong), tobacco in moderation.

In small quantities :—Tomatoes, beans, peas and other pulses, butter, cheese, ghee.

Forbidden :—Rich foods, animal foods, pastry, jellies, sugar, mushrooms, pickles, spices, confections, all acid fruits, all liquors.

**General Directions :—**

1. Moderation in animal foods, liberality in vegetables; the proportion of these must be adapted to each case.
2. Abundant fluid, of which plain hot water night and morning may form an important part.

3. Regular exercise. A gouty patient should walk daily not less than from three to four miles, unless there be reason to the contrary in the individual case. Gout, however, is not uncommon in those who take exercise freely, and the degree and kind of exercise must be carefully prescribed in each case.
4. Warm baths, tepid or cold sponging, skin friction and massage.
5. Free action of the skin, kidneys, and bowels, regular hours; warm clothing, and the avoidance of fatigue are essential.
6. Not less than seven, nor more than eight hours' sleep. The patient should go to bed early and get up early.

### NEPHRITIS—See Albuminuria.

### OBESITY.

Allowed:—Wheat, bajri, joar (in small quantity), mung water, butter (in moderation), water hot or cold (plentifully), milk (skimmed), fruits, *i.e.*, grapes, oranges; green vegetables, as cauliflower, cabbage, tomatoes, etc.

Forbidden:—Ghee, thick pulses, rice, sago, potatoes, pastry and sweets, cream, milk (except in moderation), sugar.

**General Directions :—**

1. An active life with full occupation, short hours of sleep, and the most vigorous exercise, compatible with the physical condition. Cycling, horse exercise, and fencing are especially valuable, but the form and amount of exercise must be carefully adapted to each case.
2. Free action of the bowels and skin, with regular vapour baths.

### PHTHISIS.

The diet, as to quantity and quality, and as to time, frequency, and method of administration, must necessarily vary widely according to the stage of the disease and the condition of the appetite and of the digestion.

Allowed:—All meat essences and juices; eggs preferably raw; fish; mung, wheat, rice, chana; all products of she goat—(meat, butter, ghee, milk), cream, milk, all fruits, all vegetables in moderate quantities, Drakshasara.

Forbidden:—Jamboola, Kulatha, Masha, Shimbi, hard or salt meat, re-cooked food, pickles.

**General Directions :—**

The method of feeding in phthisis is as important as the quantity and quality of food. All food should be appetisingly cooked and daintily served. The greatest variation possible even in matter of serving milk should be introduced.

1. On waking, milk, hot or warm, gradually increasing in quantity till 10 to 12 ounces are taken.
2. If preferred, there may be given as a morning stimulant, a cup of tea made with milk instead of water.
3. After one hour, substantial breakfast should be taken in bed.

4. One hour and a half after breakfast, one raw egg or two if possible broken into a glass and swallowed whole with pepper and salt or meat. To those who do not take animal food, milk may be served again.

5. Midday, a substantial meal with Draksharasa.

6. One hour and a half after midday meal, milk, raw eggs or raw meat.

7. In the afternoon tea made with milk, or milk, and abundant roti and butter.

8. At 7-30 or 8 p.m., a substantial meal.

9. At bed time milk, and if possible a raw egg in it or with it.

10. Every hour possible should be spent in airy, sunny rooms, or in the open air, and sunshine.

11. All rooms should be bright and kept well-ventilated day and night.

12. Clothing should be light and loose. It should be woollen, night and day, winter and summer. The boots should be kept thick and sound, to keep the feet not only dry, but warm.

13. Every night, the whole body should be sponged with warm water, followed by friction with a rough towel. The regular, long-continued attention to the action of the skin forms one of the most important factors in the hygienic treatment of phthisis. It should be carried out in a warm room under conditions which prevent chill. When there are night sweats, it may be necessary to regularly precede the skin friction by a soap and water cleansing.

14. Regular exercise, carefully adapted to each case; regular hours and avoidance of fatigue.

**Note** :—Generally, purgatives should not be prescribed. Sexual intercourse should be strictly forbidden..

### RHEUMATISM (Acute).

Allowed :—I. During the stage of fever and joint inflammation, fluids only, milk, milk diluted with lime-water, fruit jellies, mung water, weak China tea. The patient may be allowed to partake freely of a drink prepared by mixing a pint of milk with a pint of boiled water, adding 30 to 40 grs. of sodium bicarbonate and 10 to 20 grs. of common salt, and cooling with a lump of ice.

II. After the febrile stage is over; mung water, milk, and vegetables may be given.

III. 10 to 14 days after the temperature is normal: roti rice, sago-pudding, green vegetables generally, milk, acid fruits, tea, water of mung and other pulses.

**Note** :—Nitrogenous foods are to be taken in moderation.

Forbidden :—Pastry, sugar, sweets, potatoes; all starchy and sugary substances, except as allowed; alcohol.

### TYPHOID FEVER.

During the febrile stage: Fluids only, consisting chiefly of milk, of which at least three pints should be taken in 24 hours. The feeds should be given every two hours, one or two feeds being omitted when the patient is asleep. The milk may be diluted with water, sodawater, limewater, barley-water, or rice water.

When the milk is not digested or tympanitis is present, whey may be substituted.

After the temperature is normal for ten to fourteen days, solids may be added.

All food given in typhoid fever should be so dilute as to remain liquid in the intestines. Milk may, with advantage, be diluted with twice the quantity of water. Pure water may be given with advantage.

## POISONS AND THEIR ANTIDOTES.

The treatment of cases of poisoning, requires great care and judgment and calls for the excercise of the utmost discretion.

First consider, whether an emetic should be given. In the majority of cases, this is the correct course to follow. When the poison is an acid or other corrosive agent, however, its action on the membrane of the stomach and the aesophagus may have been such as to render the use of an emetic highly dangerous from the liability to perforation. The proper course then is to neutralise the acid or corrosive agent and not to attempt its removal.

It is important to find the approximate quantity of the poison, which has been taken, in order that the needful quantity of the antidote may be judged.

Emetics—(1) Mustard and water; a tablespoonful in 8 oz. of warm water.

(2) Common salt 2 tablespoonfuls in 8 oz. tepid water.

(3) Madan phala, with water.

(4) Madanadivaman 30 grs. in 4 oz. tepid water.

(5) Copper sulphate (Tutha tikadi) 5 to 10 grs. in 4 oz. of warm water.

(6) Arkachurna 4 grs. in 4 oz. warm water.

If none of the above remedies be immediately available copious draughts of warm water and tickling the back of the throat should be tried.

The treatment to follow the emetic (if administered), will require quick but careful consideration. The patient's general condition must be carefully observed; and every means taken to increase the resistance to the poison, until its effects have passed off. Cardiac stimulants may be required; while artificial respiration and warmth are most important.

The following are the antidotes described against various poisons:—

**Arsenic and its preparations** (Acute poisoning).

Emetic. The complete removal of contents is important.

Dialysed iron, one tablespoonful followed by a little common salt in a tablespoonful of water; repeat frequently until ten doses have been taken, or Ferric Hydrate.

If neither of the foregoing be available, give large quantities of calcined magnesia mixed with wâter to form a thin paste.

Milk and ghee.

Sesamum oil ½ pint in 1 pint of water.

Iced barley water for thirst; stimulants. Hot water bottles to extremities.

**Copper salts.**

Vomiting usually occurs in cases of poisoning by copper salts. When this is not the case, remedies 1 and 2 should be used.

(1) Before emptying stomach, give large quantities of milk and ghee.

(2) Emetic.

(3) Demulcent drinks, e. g., Isapghul water, &c.

**Lead and salts** (Acute poisoning).

(1) Emetic.

(2) Give Samudrak virechana ½ oz. in a tumblerful of water.

(3) Milk, ghee or demulcent drinks.

**Mercury and salts** (Acute poisoning) corrosive sublimate cinnabar.

(1) Do not empty stomach before giving large quantities of ghee; and milk or flour and water.

(2) Emetic.

(3) For pain and purging, opium 1 gr. in 1 oz. of water

(4) Stimulants and demulcents, if much depression.

**Zinc salts.**

Do not use emetic. But give :—

(1) Large draughts of ghee and milk.

(2) Large quantities of sodium carbonate and Potassium carbonate dissolved in warm water.

(3) Triphala and strong tea.

(4) Demulcents.

(5) For pain, 1½ grs. opium with 1 oz. of water.

**Aconite.**

Emetic.

Lay the patient fiat.

Stimulants. Warmth to extremities.

Artificial respiration and friction.

Recumbent position to be maintained.

**Croton oil** and **Violent purgatives.**

Emetic.

Demulcent drinks, milk and ghee.

Relieve pain by ½ gr. opium in 1 oz. of water.

Stimulants.

**Opium.**

Emetic.

Hot coffee.

Rouse patient and dash cold water on face.

Warmth to extremities.

Artificial respiration.

**Nux Vomica.**

Emetic.

Samudraka virechana 1 oz. as a purgative in half a tumblerful of water.

Demulcent drinks.

**Datura.**

Emetic. Large doses of Trifala.

Hot tea and coffee. Afterwards, give purgatives. Give warmth to the body. Artificial respiration; keep the patient awake.

**Indian Hemp.**

Emetics. Purgatives. Give stimulants such as tea, coffee, &c. Treat symptoms. Keep the patient awake.

**Note.**—The antidotes here given are those which are more generally available and which may be used, pending the arrival of expert assistance. The treatment by stomach tube or hypodermic injections, etc., which requires expert knowledge, has been purposely omitted

## THE PULSE RATE.

In health, the pulse rate varies widely according to a number of conditions. The pulse is generally more frequent in females than in males; during and after exertion, unless long continued; during digestion or mental excitement, also more frequent in the morning than later in the day. It is temporarily accelerated after a sudden change of posture from the recumbent to the sitting, and from either to the standing position, especially during convalescence; and in other states, where the action of the heart is feeble.

The relation of the respiration rate to the pulse rate may broadly be expressed as about 1 to

| Ages. | | Beats per minute. |
|---|---|---|
| In the fœtus in utero | .. ..Between | 150 & 140 |
| In new-born infants | .. .. ,, | 140 & 130 |
| During first year . | .. ..From | 130 to 115 |
| During second year | .. .. ,, | 115 to 100 |
| During third year | .. .. ,, | 105 to 95 |
| From 3 to 7 .. | .. .. ,, | 100 to 90 |
| ,, 7 to 14 .. | .. .. ,, | 90 to 75 |
| ,, 14 to 21 .. | .. .. ,, | 85 to 75 |
| ,, 21 to 65 .. | .. .. ,, | 75 to 65 |
| In old age.. .. | .. ..Between | 85 & 75 |

## RESPIRATION.

| | |
|---|---|
| Two months to two years .. .. .. | 35 per minute. |
| Two to six years . .. .. .. | 23 „ |
| Six to twelve years .. .. .. | 20 „ |
| Twelve to fifteen years .. .. .. | 18 „ |
| Fifteen to twenty-one years .. .. | 16 to 18 „ |

Respiration in the adult female is usually slightly more rapid than in the male; especially during pregnancy.

## TEMPERATURE.

The average in health is 98.4°F.

It is normally one degree higher under the tongue than in the axilla, and nearly that in the vagina and the rectum. It is highest upon awaking in the morning and lowest at midnight; the daily range rarely exceeds 1.8°F. above or below the average.

The axillary temperature may fall to 97°F. without collapse or rise to 100°F. without indicating febrile disturbance. A rise of one degree usually marks an increase of the pulse from six to 10 beats per minute.

Continued temperature above 98.4°F. indicates a pathological condition; 103° to 105° severe fever; 105° to 108° danger; 108° to 109° impending death. This does not imply, however, that in an ephemeral fever, the high degree is necessarily dangerous. It sometimes happens, especially in intermittent fevers, that the temperature rises as high as 106° or 108° for a short time only, which rise must be considered idiosyncratic, rather than pathological. A temperature of 104° is generally alarming in acute rheumatism, and may cause cardiac complications. In jaundice a rise of temperature is unfavourable. A rise of temperature in tuberculosis shows an advance of the disease or the incidence of complications.

## MEASURE FOR FLUIDS.

60 minims = 1 Drachm.
8 drachms = 1 Ounce.
20 Ounces = 1 Pint.
8 Pints = 1 Gallon.

1 Teaspoonful = 1 Drachm.
1 Tablespoonful = 4 „ or ½ oz.

# AXIOMS ABOUT MEDICINES.

## TABLE OF INDIAN AND ENGLISH WEIGHTS.

| | | | | | |
|---|---|---|---|---|---|
| 1 Gunja | = .... | = .. | .. | 1⅞grs. = | |
| 6 Gunjas | 1 Masha | .. | .. | 11¼ „ | 1/16 Tola |
| 4 Masha | 1 Shana | .. | .. | 45 „ | ¼ „ |
| 2 Shanas | 1 Kola | .. | .. | 90 „ | ½ „ |
| 2 Kolas | 1 Karsha | .. | .. | 180 „ | 1 „ |
| 2 Karsha | 1 Shukti | .. | .. | 360 „ | 2 „ |
| 2 Shukti | 1 Pala | .. | 1oz. | 282½ „ | 4 „ |
| 2 Pala | 1 Prasriti | .. | 3 „ | 127½ „ | 8 „ |
| 2 Prasriti | 1 Kudava | .. | 6 „ | 255 „ | 16 „ |
| 2 Kudava | 1 Sharava | .. | 18 „ | 72½ „ | 32 „ |
| 2 Sharava | 1 Prastha | 1lb | 10 „ | 145 „ | 64 „ |
| 100 Pala | 1 Tula | 10 „ | 4 „ | 250 „ | 400 „ |
| 4 Prastha | 1 Adhaka | 6 „ | 9 „ | 142½ „ | 256 „ |
| 4 Adhaka | 1 Drona | 26 „ | 5 „ | 132½ „ | 1024 „ |
| 2 Dronas | 1 Shoorpa | 52 „ | 10 „ | 265 „ | 2048 „ |
| 2000 Palas | 1 Bhara | 205 „ | 11 „ | 187½ „ | 8000 „ |

Note :— 1⅞ grains = 1 Gunja | 437½ grains = 1 oz.
180 „ = 1 Tola | 7000 „ = 1 lb.

## DOSES PROPORTIONATE TO AGE.

If the adult dose of any given drug, be 24 grs. or about 13 Gunjas,
a patient under 6 months old, would take 1 gr. or ½ Gunja.

| | | | | | | | |
|---|---|---|---|---|---|---|---|
| Under | ½ year to | 1 year | would take | 1½ gr. | or | ¾ Gunja | |
| From | 1 „ | 2 „ | „ | 2 „ | | 1 | „ |
| „ | 2 „ | 3 „ | „ | 3 „ | | 1½ | „ |
| „ | 3 „ | 4 „ | „ | 4 „ | | 2 | „ |
| „ | 4 „ | 6 „ | „ | 6 „ | | 3 | „ |
| „ | 6 „ | 10 „ | „ | 8 „ | | 4 | „ |
| „ | 10 „ | 13 „ | „ | 10 „ | | 5 | „ |
| „ | 13 „ | 16 „ | „ | 12 „ | | 6 | „ |
| „ | 16 „ | 18 „ | „ | 16 „ | | 8½ | „ |
| „ | 18 „ | 20 „ | „ | 20 „ | | 10½ | „ |
| „ | 21 „ | .. | | 24 „ | | 13 | „ |

The proportionate dose for any age, twenty years or less, may also be found by taking one-twentieth of the full therapeutic dose, and multiplying the result by the age in years.

The doses may require lessening for patients advanced in life, but no exact rules can be laid down.

## SOME AXIOMS ABOUT ADMINISTRATION OF MEDICINES.

The action of medicines is modified by sex, age, temperament, and diathesis, idiosyncrasies, habits of life; race and mental impressions. Women being possessed of more delicate organisations than men, rarely require the same doses. Avoid **aloes** during pregnancy and **mercury** during anæmic chlorosis.

Old age and childhood do not bear doses, proportionately to manhood youth. Excepting under urgent circumstances, an **opiate** should never be administered to an infant. While mercury is better borne in childhood and old age, than in middle life. Inquire always as to indiosyncrasies, especially towards mercury and opium.

**Town dwellers** particularly, in overcrowded quarters, cannot bear doses which are quite suitable for those of rural or outdoor life. Mark this as to children especially.

**Passions** and **affections** of the mind markedly influence the action of remedies, especially narcotics. **Faith** in the prescription or in the prescriber, may remove mountains of difficulties. Every means should be used to implant confidence and stimulate hope.

**The doses** of any given medicine, particularly a narcotic or purgative, should be regulated in accordance with the effect produced in each individual, rather than with published tables; the latter are given as guides merely and are not infallible. The character, period and form of disease influence the operations of medicines in no slight degree. In epidemics it is worthy of note, that a remedy which is highly beneficial at one period, appears to possess no efficacy at another. Usually, while, the onset and climax of an epidemic are marked by numerous deaths, with its wane recoveries are the rule; hence the period of an epidemic influence the action of medicines.

**Diet** exercises a marked influence, Antiphlogistics (medicines that subdue inflammation or fever), refuse to act in the presence of an excess of animal foods along with stimulants; and the latter notoriously interfere with the action of mercurials; and iron salts are inoperative, when confronted with vegetable acids during febrile conditions.

The **time of administration** affects the action of medicines. Narcotics, emetics and diaphoretics operate most favourably when administered an hour or two before bed time. Diuretics are best given during the day, when the body may be kept cool. Resinous cathartics are best at bed time; other cathartics such as neutral salts, oil, and those whose operation is speedy, early in the morning. Arsenic acts best on a full stomach.

**Light, air** and **exercise** possess great therapeutic power, and are very essential adjutants to drugs. Confinement in close, dark, ill-ventilated apartments, counteracts any benefit that might be had from tonics, and violent physical action retards the effect of diuretics.

**Season** also is a modifying agent; some diseases independent of remedial measures, improve at certain season, and relapse at others; tuberculous patients almost invariably improve in summer, remain stationary in winter, and decline in spring.

# INDEX OF DISEASES.

*Arranged according to Sanskrit Alphabets.*

## Index of Diseases.

*Arranged according to Sanskrit Alphabets.*

## Index of Diseases

*Arranged according to Sanskrit Alphabets,*



# INDEX OF MEDICINES.

*Arranged according to Sanskrit Alphabets.*

## Index of Medicines.

*Arranged according to Sanskrit Alphabets.*

## Index of Medicines.

*Arranged according to Sanskrit Alphabets.*

## Index of Medicines

*Arranged according to Sanskrit Alphabets.*

## Index of Medicines.

*Arranged according to Sanskrit Alphabets.*

## Index of Medicines.

*Arranged according to Sanskrit Alphabets.*

# ERRATA.

| *Page.* | *Line.* | *Incorrect.* | *Correct.* |
|---|---|---|---|
| 120 | 27 | $\frac{1}{8}$ gr. | 1/64 gr. |
| 128 | 11 | Chandana | Chandana Oil. |
| 132 | 1 | Santonine | Butea Seeds. |
| 131 | 36 | Empty Stomach. | Three times a day for three days followed, &c. |
| 157 | 28 | 1/20 gr. Croton Seeds. | 1/10 gr. Shudha Croton Seeds. |
| 157 | 26 | 1/5 gr. " " | $\frac{1}{3}$ gr. " " |
| 165 | 5 | $\frac{1}{3}$ gr. " " | $\frac{1}{2}$ gr. " " |
| 167 | 7 | 1 gr. Datura Seeds | $\frac{1}{8}$ gr. Datura Seeds. |
| 167 | 7 | 1 gr. Aconite | 1/18 gr. Aconite. |